Practice Test #1

Reading

DIRECTIONS: The reading practice test you are about to take is multiple-choice with only one correct answer per question. Read each test item and circle your answer on the answer sheet below. When you have completed the practice test, you may check your answers with the answers on the answer key following the test.

Answer Sheet

1.	a	b	c	d		21.	a	b	c	d
2.	a	b	c	d		22.	a	b	c	d
3.	a	b	c	d		23.	a	b	c	d
4.	a	b	c	d		24.	a	b	c	d
5.	a	b	c	d		25.	a	b	c	d
6.	a	b	c	d		26.	a	b	c	d
7.	a	b	c	d		27.	a	b	c	d
8.	a	b	c	d		28.	a	b	c	d
9.	a	b	c	d		29.	a	b	c	d
10.	a	b	c	d		30.	a	b	c	d
11.	a	b	c	d		31.	a	b	c	d
12.	a	b	c	d		32.	a	b	c	d
13.	a	b	c	d		33.	a	b	c	d
14.	a	b	c	d		34.	a	b	c	d
15.	a	b	c	d		35.	a	b	c	d
16.	a	b	c	d		36.	a	b	c	d
17.	a	b	c	d		37.	a	b	c	d
18.	a	b	c	d		38.	a	b	c	d
19.	a	b	c	d		39.	a	b	c	d
20.	a	b	c	d		40.	a	b	c	d

Reading Test

Read the passage below and answer questions 1-5.

Chang-Rae Lee's debut and award-winning novel <u>Native Speaker</u> is about Henry Park, a Korean-American individual who struggles to find his place as an immigrant in a suburb of New York City. This novel addresses the notion that as the individuals who know us best, our family, peers, and lovers are the individuals who direct our lives and end up defining us. Henry Park is confronted with this reality in the very beginning of the novel, which begins:

The day my wife left she gave me a list of who I was.

Upon separating from his wife, Park struggles with racial and ethnic identity issues due to his loneliness. Through Parks' work as an undercover operative for a private intelligence agency, the author presents the theme of espionage as metaphor for the internal divide that Park experiences as an immigrant. This dual reality creates two worlds for Park and increases his sense of uncertainty with regard to his place in society. While he constantly feels like an outsider looking in, he also feels like he belongs to neither world.

Chang-Rae Lee is also a first-generation Korean American immigrant. He immigrated to America at the early age of three. Themes of identity, race, and cultural alienation pervade his works. His interests in these themes no doubt stem from his first-hand experience as a kid growing up in a Korean household while going to an American school. Lee is also author of <u>A Gesture Life</u> and <u>Aloft</u>. The protagonists are similar in that they deal with labels placed on them based on race, color, and language. Consequently, all of these characters struggle to belong in America.

Lee's novels address differences within a nation's mix of race, religion, and history, and the necessity of assimilation between cultures. In his works and through his characters, Lee shows us both the difficulties and the subtleties of the immigrant experience in America. He urges us to consider the role of borders and to consider why the idea of opening up one's borders is so frightening. In an ever-changing world in which cultures are becoming more intermingled, the meaning of identity must be constantly redefined, especially when the security of belonging to a place is becoming increasingly elusive. As our world grows smaller with increasing technological advances, these themes in Lee's novels become even more pertinent.

1. Which of the following best describes the purpose of this passage?
    a. to criticize
    b. to analyze
    c. to entertain
    d. to inform

2. Why does the author of the passage quote the first line of the novel <u>Native Speaker</u>?
    a. to illustrate one of the themes in the novel
    b. to show how the book is semi-autobiographical
    c. it is the main idea of the novel
    d. to create interest in the novel

3. According to the passage, which of the following is *not* a main theme of Lee's novels?
    a. identity
    b. culture
    c. immigration
    d. espionage

4. Based on the passage, why do Lee's novels focus on race and cultural identity?
    a. because Lee was born in Korea
    b. because Lee's ancestors are Korean
    c. because Lee immigrated to America at a young age
    d. because Lee feels these issues are the biggest problem facing America

5. How does the author of the passage feel about the ideas presented in Lee's novels?
    a. concerned about the disappearance of cultures in a rapidly expanding and mixed world
    b. excited that immigrants are easily able to redefine and establish themselves in new cultures
    c. certain that all borders will eventually be eliminated so world cultures will commingle and fully assimilate
    d. critical regarding the role technology has played in society and how it destroys the immigrant experience

Read the set of directions below to answer questions 6-9.

This formula is for people with deficiencies and anemic conditions. It aids in the body's absorption of vital minerals such as iron, calcium, zinc, potassium, and sulfur. Take the following ingredients:

Parsley root	Comfrey root
Yellow dock	Watercress
Nettles	Kelp
Irish moss	

Slowly simmer equal parts of these herbs with four ounces to a half-quart of water. Continue to simmer slowly until the volume of liquid is reduced by half. Strain, reserve the liquid, and cover the herbs with water once more. Then simmer again for 10 minutes. Strain and combine the two liquids. Cook the liquid down until the volume is reduced by half. Add an equal amount of blackstrap molasses. Take one tablespoon four to five times daily, not exceeding four tablespoons in a 24-hour period.

6. What is the main reason for taking this formula?
   a. to serve as a mineral supplement
   b. to get rid of unnecessary minerals
   c. to reduce the absorption of minerals
   d. to increase the absorption of minerals

7. If a ¼ ounce of yellow dock is used, how much watercress should be used?
   a. ½ ounce
   b. ¼ ounce
   c. ⅓ ounce
   d. 1 ounce

8. If a patient follows the directions correctly, how often could the medicine be taken?
   a. once every two hours
   b. once every four hours
   c. once every three hours
   d. once every six hours

9. Which cooking process is *not* required to make this formula?
   a. evaporating
   b. filtering
   c. whisking
   d. mixing

Use the data in the table below to answer question 10-14.

Precipitation (inches)			
Date	Albany	Coral Bay	Bunbury
6/1	0.01	0.02	0.02
6/2	0.25	0.35	0.00
6/3	0.55	0.75	0.20
6/4	0.00	0.45	0.10
6/5	0.90	1.01	0.50
6/6	2.00	2.15	1.90
6/7	0.95	1.05	1.15

10. How much more rain did Albany receive than Bunbury on the third of the month?
    a. 0.30 inches
    b. 0.35 inches
    c. 0.55 inches
    d. 0.25 inches

11. What was the average amount of precipitation received in all areas on the fifth of the month?
    a. 0.80 inches
    b. 1.01 inches
    c. 2.41 inches
    d. 0.95 inches

12. On what day was flooding most likely the greatest concern?
    a. first
    b. fifth
    c. sixth
    d. seventh

13. Based on the data in the table, which city has the driest climate?
    a. Albany
    b. Coral Bay
    c. Bunbury
    d. They all have the same climate.

14. Which statement best compares the precipitation between Albany and Coral Bay?
    a. Albany is usually slightly wetter than Coral Bay.
    b. Coral Bay is usually slightly wetter than Albany.
    c. Coral Bay is always much wetter than Albany.
    d. There is no difference between Albany and Coral Bay.

Read the paragraph below to answer questions 15-17.

> The Channel Tunnel is an underwater tunnel that passes through the English Channel and connects England and France. Work on the Tunnel began in 1987 despite much controversy. Many protests took place due to concerns for the environment, fears about terrorism, and the risk of fire. Construction required five thousand workers to dig undersea in the Channel at all hours of the day using laser-guided Tunnel Boring machines. These machines cost around 7.5 million pounds and could construct up to one thousand meters of tunnel a month. Two tunnels were built for passenger trains, with a smaller service tunnel was built in between for maintenance and an escape route in the case of emergency. Costs to construct the Tunnel were much higher than anticipated, and loans were required to finance its construction. After many delays and additional costs, the tunnel was finally opened in 1995. The concrete tunnel's overall length is 50 kilometers, with 40 km being undersea. The journey time from England to France is only 35 minutes, and trains run every 20 minutes. Travel between London and Brussels takes three hours and 10 minutes. In its first year of service, the Tunnel accounted for 40% of the traffic across the Channel and had a turnover of 299 million pounds. Nonetheless, it suffered a huge loss of 925 million pounds due to the high interest the Tunnel company had to pay on the 8.1 billion pounds borrowed from banks.

15. Given that one Tunnel Boring machine could build 1,000 m of tunnel a month and the Tunnel is 50 km long, how fast could the Tunnel have been built using two Tunnel Boring machines if there had been no delays?
    a. just under 5 years
    b. about 1 year
    c. just over 4 years
    d. just over 2 years

16. If a passenger leaves London on the 8:35 a.m. train, what is their expected arrival time in Brussels? (note: Brussels is one time zone east of London)
    a. 9:55 a.m.
    b. 10:10 a.m.
    c. 12:45 p.m.
    d. 1:10 p.m.

17. According to the passage, what was *not* a reason people were against the construction of the Tunnel?
    a. It will disrupt and pollute marine habitats.
    b. It will take too long to build.
    c. Fires will endanger people and the environment.
    d. It will threaten national security.

For each of the words below, pick the answer choice that most closely means the same thing.

18. vehement
    a. troubled
    b. intense
    c. changeable
    d. obstinate

19. diatribe
    a. criticism
    b. apology
    c. commend
    d. merit

20. cogitate
    a. surprise
    b. endanger
    c. confuse
    d. deliberate

21. invidious
    a. offensive
    b. pleasant
    c. ornate
    d. infectious

22. hyperbole
    a. reference
    b. amendment
    c. exaggeration
    d. demarcation

23. innocuous
    a. harmful
    b. innocent
    c. scandalous
    d. hidden

Answer questions 24 – 28 based on the debate below.

> *Forest Manager:* Salvage logging is the removal of dead or dying forest stands left behind by a fire or disease. It has been practiced for several decades. Dead or dying trees become fuel that feeds future fires. The best way to minimize the risk of forest fires is to remove the dead timber from the forest floor. Salvage logging followed by replanting ensures the reestablishment of desirable tree species. For instance, planting conifers accelerates the return of fire resistant forests. Harvesting timber benefits forests by reducing fuel load, thinning the forest stands, and relieving competition between trees. Burned landscapes leave behind black surfaces and ash layers that result in very high soil temperatures. These high soil temperatures can kill many plant species. Logging mixes the soil, thereby decreasing surface temperatures to more normal levels. Shade from small, woody material left behind by logging also helps to decrease surface temperatures. After an area has been salvage logged, seedlings in the area begin to regenerate almost immediately; nonetheless, regeneration can take several years in unmanaged areas.
>
> *Ecology professor:* Salvage logging transfers material like small, broken branches to the forest floor where it is available for fuel. The removal of larger, less flammable trees while leaving behind small dead limbs increases the risk of forest fires. In unmanaged areas, these woody materials are found more commonly on the tops of trees where they are unavailable to fires. Logging destroys old growth forests more resistant to wildfires and creates younger forests more vulnerable to severe fires. In old growth forests, branches of bigger trees are higher above the floor where fires may not reach. Replanting after wildfires creates monoculture plantations in which only a single crop is planted and produced. This monoculture creates less biological diversity and less disease resistant vegetation that in turn increases vulnerability to fire. Salvage logging also interferes with natural forest regeneration by killing most of the seedlings that reemerge on their own after a wildfire. It disrupts the soil, increases erosion, and removes most of the shade needed for young seedlings to grow.

24. According to the professor, how are unmanaged areas advantageous in distributing small, woody materials after a fire?
    a. They are left on the forest floor and provide nutrients to the soil.
    b. They are left on the forest floor and serve as fuel for fires.
    c. They are left on the tops of trees where fires cannot reach.
    d. They are distributed more evenly across the forest floor.

25. A study compared two plots of land that were managed differently after a fire. Plot A was salvage logged, while Plot B was left unmanaged. When a second fire occurred, they compared two plant groups between Plots A and B and found that both plant groups burned with greater severity in Plot A than in Plot B. Which viewpoint do these results support?
    only the manager
    only the professor
    both the manager and professor
    neither the manager nor the professor

26. What is the main idea of the forest manager's argument?
    a. Salvage logging is beneficial because it removes dead or dying timber from the forest floor, thereby reducing the risk of future fires.
    b. Salvage logging is beneficial because it has been practiced for several decades.
    c. Salvage logging is harmful because it raises soil temperatures above normal levels and threatens the health of plant species.
    d. Salvage logging is beneficial because it provides shade for seedlings to grow after a wildfire.

27. According to the professor, young forests are more vulnerable to severe fires than old growth forests. Which of the following statements does *not* support this view?
    a. In younger forests, small branches are closer to the forest floor and more available for fires.
    b. Old growth forests contain larger and taller trees, where branches are high up and fires may not reach.
    c. Younger forests have less biological diversity and less disease-resistant trees.
    d. Larger trees common in old growth forests serve as the main fuel source for severe fires.

28. Whose viewpoints would be validated by a future study looking at the distribution and regeneration of seedlings for several years following a wildfire in both managed and unmanaged forests?
    a. only the manager
    b. only the professor
    c. both the manager and professor
    d. neither the manager nor professor

Use the passage below to answer questions 29-33.

During the 1800s, Charles Darwin became known for his studies of plants and animals on the Galapagos Islands. He is often referred to as "the father of evolution," because he was first to describe a mechanism by which organisms change over time.

The Galapagos Islands are situated off the coast of South America. Much of Darwin's work on the islands focused on the birds. He noticed that island birds looked similar to finches on the South American continent and resembled a type of modified finch. The only differences in the finches Darwin saw were in their beaks and the kind of food they ate. Finches on the mainland were seed-eating birds, but the island finches ate insects, seeds, plant matter, egg yolks, and blood.

Darwin theorized that the island finches were offspring of one type of mainland finch. The population of finches was changing over time due to their environment. He believed the finches' eating habits changed because of the island's limited food supply. As the finches began to eat differently, the way their beaks worked and looked changed as well. For instance, insect-eating finches needed longer beaks for digging in the ground. Seed-eating and nut-eating finches required thicker beaks to crack the seed shells.

The process by which the finches changed happened over many generations. Among the population of beetle-eating finches, those finches born with longer, sharper beaks naturally had access to more beetles than those finches with shorter beaks. As a result, the sharp-beaked, insect-eating finches thrived and produced many offspring, while the short-beaked insect-eating finches gradually died out. The sharp beak was in effect selected by nature to thrive. The same thing happened in each finch population until finches within the same population began to look similar to each other and different from finches of other populations. These observations eventually led Darwin to develop the theory of natural selection.

29. Why is Charles Darwin called "the father of evolution?"
    a. because he coined the term "evolution"
    b. because he was the first scientist to study species on the Galapagos Islands
    c. because he was the first to describe how organisms changed over time
    d. because he was the first to suggest that birds adapted to their environment

30. What is the main point of this passage?
    a. to inform
    b. to entertain
    c. to critique
    d. to persuade

31. According to the passage, why did finches with sharp, long beaks thrive while other finches died off?
    a. They were able to reproduce faster than other types of finches on the island.
    b. They were more numerous and eventually outlived the other finches on the island.
    c. They were randomly selected by nature to reproduce over other types of finches on the island.
    d. They had better access to insects than other types of finches on the island.

32. Based on Darwin's studies on the islands, what could also be inferred about how geography affects the diversity of species?
    a. Geographical barriers decrease diversity of a species.
    b. Geographical barriers increase diversity of a species.
    c. Geographical barriers have an insignificant impact on the diversity of a species.
    d. There is no relationship between geographical barriers and the diversity of a species.

33. Which of the following statements correctly compares the finches Darwin observed in the Galapagos Islands with the finches found on the mainland?
    a. The island finches were very similar with no visible differences.
    b. The island finches differed only in the shape of their beaks.
    c. The island finches differed only in size.
    d. The island finches differed in the shape of their beaks and their diet.

Answer questions 34 through 36 based on the paragraph below.

The Australian town of Bundanoon recently placed a ban on all bottled water to reduce carbon dioxide emissions associated with bottling and transporting the water. Kingston, a local businessman, organized a campaign group called "Bundy on Tap." The group held a vote at the town's Memorial Hall, where 400 people voted in favor of the ban with only two dissenting votes. Free water fountains will be installed across town in an effort to replace bottled water. Ghent, a city in Brussels, has elected Thursdays as "meatless days." Everyone will eat strictly vegetarian meals in an effort to improve overall health and reduce the environmental impact of raising livestock, an industry that accounts for 18 percent of global greenhouse gas emissions. City-financed schools say they will offer only vegetarian meals on the menu on Thursdays.

34. Why do residents of Bundanoon want to ban bottled water?
    a. They want to decrease emissions produced from the bottling and shipping of water.
    b. They want to install water fountains all over town instead of having to buy bottled water.
    c. They want to save on costs associated with bottling and transporting water.
    d. They want to help conserve water due to an increasingly limited supply.

35. Why do residents of Ghent want to restrict the amount of meat consumed by the population?
    a. because the population is obese
    b. because the livestock industry contributes a large amount to greenhouse gases
    c. because they want to support city-financed schools and help them save money
    d. because they are concerned about the treatment of animals

36. Which statement best describes the vote held in Bundanoon over the elimination of bottled water?
    a. The majority is slightly in favor.
    b. They are equally in favor and in opposition.
    c. The majority is in opposition.
    d. The majority is in favor.

Use the information in the table below to answer question 37 – 40.

Information on Hiking Trails in the Area			
Trail	**Length**	**Level of Difficulty**	**Attractions**
1. Beaverton Falls	2.6 miles	Easy	Three waterfalls with picnic areas open May-September; trail is suitable for all ages. End of trail connects to Copper Creek Trail.
2. Silver Bullet	5.5 miles	Easy – Moderate	Follows the Salmon River; fishing allowed July-October. Meets the Toulanne River and connects to the Toulanne Trail.
3. Eagle Eye	8.2 miles	Moderate – Hard	Trail has steep terrain, narrow segments, and switchbacks. Features two waterfalls and excellent panoramic views at the ridge
4. Toulanne	7.5 miles	Moderate	Beautiful rock formations along trail, with close views of canyon walls and Toulanne River. Boat rentals April-November
5. Copper Creek	9.5 miles	Hard	Icy in winter, and many areas require climbing gear. Caving and climbing gear rentals available year-round.

37. Which trail does not connect to another trail?
    a. Beaverton Falls
    b. Silver Bullet
    c. Eagle Eye
    d. Copper Creek

38. This summer the Esperanza family is planning to have their family reunion outdoors surrounded by beautiful scenery. People of all ages are expected to attend. Which trail would be best for them to use?
    a. Beaverton Falls
    b. Eagle Eye
    c. Toulanne
    d. Copper Creek

39. The Cornell family wants to do some fishing in June. Which trail should they choose?
    a. Beaverton Falls
    b. Eagle Eye
    c. Copper Creek
    d. Toulanne

40. If Joey and Katrina hike an average of 3 miles per hour, about how long will it take them if they take the Beaverton Falls trail and follow it through the Copper Creek trail?
    a. 3 hours
    b. 3 ½ hours
    c. 4 hours
    d. 4 ½ hours

Mathematics

DIRECTIONS: The mathematics practice test you are about to take is multiple-choice with only one correct answer per question. Read each test item and circle your answer on the answer sheet below. When you have completed the practice test, you may check your answers with the answers on the answer key following the test.

Answer Sheet

1.	a	b	c	d		24.	a	b	c	d
2.	a	b	c	d		25.	a	b	c	d
3.	a	b	c	d		26.	a	b	c	d
4.	a	b	c	d		27.	a	b	c	d
5.	a	b	c	d		28.	a	b	c	d
6.	a	b	c	d		29.	a	b	c	d
7.	a	b	c	d		30.	a	b	c	d
8.	a	b	c	d		31.	a	b	c	d
9.	a	b	c	d		32.	a	b	c	d
10.	a	b	c	d		33.	a	b	c	d
11.	a	b	c	d		34.	a	b	c	d
12.	a	b	c	d		35.	a	b	c	d
13.	a	b	c	d		36.	a	b	c	d
14.	a	b	c	d		37.	a	b	c	d
15.	a	b	c	d		38.	a	b	c	d
16.	a	b	c	d		39.	a	b	c	d
17.	a	b	c	d		40.	a	b	c	d
18.	a	b	c	d		41.	a	b	c	d
19.	a	b	c	d		42.	a	b	c	d
20.	a	b	c	d		43.	a	b	c	d
21.	a	b	c	d		44.	a	b	c	d
22.	a	b	c	d		45.	a	b	c	d
23.	a	b	c	d						

Mathematics Test

1. If Sara can read 15 pages in 10 minutes, how long will it take her to read 45 pages?
    a. 20 minutes
    b. 30 minutes
    c. 40 minutes
    d. 50 minutes

2. Restaurant customers tip their server only 8 percent for poor service. If their tip was $3.70, how much was their bill?
    a. $40.15
    b. $44.60
    c. $46.25
    d. $50.45

3. If Leonard bought 2 packs of batteries for x amount of dollars, how many packs of batteries could he purchase for $5.00 at the same rate?
    a. 10x
    b. 2/x
    c. 2x
    d. 10/x

4. Choose the algebraic expression that best represents the following situation: Jeral's test score (J) was 5 points higher than half of Kara's test score (K).
    a. $J = \frac{1}{2}K + 5$
    b. $J = 2K - 5$
    c. $K = (J - \frac{1}{2}) - 5$
    d. $K = \frac{1}{2}J - 5$

5. Enrique weighs 5 pounds more than twice Brendan's weight. If their total weight is 225 pounds, how much does Enrique weigh?
    a. 125 pounds
    b. 152 pounds
    c. 115 pounds
    d. 165 pounds

6. What does $(4x - y) + (-10 + y)$ equal if $x = 3$ and $y = 4$?
    a. 2
    b. -2
    c. 22
    d. 14

7. A pasta salad was chilled in the refrigerator at 35° F overnight for 9 hours. The temperature of the pasta dish dropped from 86° F to 38° F. What was the average rate of cooling per hour?
    a. 4.8°/hr
    b. 5.3°/hr
    c. 5.15°/hr
    d. 0.532°/hr

8. Loral received all her grades for the semester (in parentheses) along with the weight for each grade, shown below. What is her final grade?

Weight
45% = 3 tests (80%, 75%, 92%)
25% = final (88%)
15% = paper (91%)
15% = 2 oral quizzes each worth 25 points (22, 18)

a. 88
b. 86
c. 79
d. 85

9. The following items were purchased at the grocery store. What was the average price paid for the items?

Item	Cost	Quantity
Milk	$3.50/carton	2
Banana	$0.30 each	5
Can of soup	$1.25/can	3
Carrots	$0.45/stick	6

a. $0.34
b. $0.55
c. $0.93
d. $1.38

10. What does 68% equal?
a. .0068
b. .68
c. 6.8
d. 6800

11. Multiply 2 1/7 x 3 2/3.
a. 4/7
b. 1 32/45
c. 7 6/7
d. 1 1/3

12. Find $(27 \div 9) \times (\sqrt{25} \times 2)$.
a. 90
b. 12
c. 45
d. 30

13. What is the missing number in the sequence: 4, 6, 10, 18, __, 66.
    a. 22
    b. 34
    c. 45
    d. 54

14. Which of the following is an improper fraction?
    a. 2/3
    b. 1 3/5
    c. 5/2
    d. 2.50

15. Convert 250 centimeters to kilometers.
    a. 0.0025 km
    b. 0.025 km
    c. 0.250 km
    d. 2.50 km

16. Rick renovated his home. He made his bedroom 40% larger (length and width) than its original size. If the original dimensions were 144 inches by 168 inches, how big is his room now if measured in feet?
    a. 12 ft x 14 ft
    b. 16.8 ft x 19.6 ft
    c. 4.8 ft x 5.6 ft
    d. 201.6 ft x 235.2 ft

17. What is $(x^2)^3 \cdot (y^2)^5 \cdot (y^4)^3$?
    a. x^6y^{22}
    b. x^6y^{120}
    c. x^5y^{14}
    d. x^6y^{-2}

18. Simplify the following fraction: $[(x^2)^5y^6z^2] / [x^4(y^3)^4z^2]$.
    a. $x^{40}\,y^{72}\,z^4$
    b. $x^6\,y^{-6}$
    c. $x^3\,y^{-1}$
    d. $x^{14}\,y^{18}\,z^4$

19. There are 64 fluid ounces in a ½ gallon. If Nora fills a tank that holds 8 ¾ gallons, how many ounces will she use?
    a. 560 ounces
    b. 1,024 ounces
    c. 1,088 ounces
    d. 1,120 ounces

20. Shaylee goes shopping for two types of fruit: mangoes that cost $2.00 each and coconuts that cost $4.00 each. If she buys 10 pieces of fruit and spends $30.00, how many pieces of each type of fruit did she buy?
   a. 4 mangoes and 6 coconuts
   b. 5 mangoes and 5 coconuts
   c. 6 mangoes and 4 coconuts
   d. 7 mangoes and 3 coconuts

Use the graph below to answer questions 21 and 22.

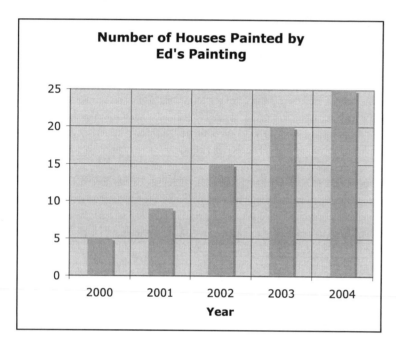

21. What is the average number of houses Ed painted each year from 2000 to 2004?
   a. 15
   b. 74
   c. 12
   d. 22

22. Assuming Ed's Painting did not experience any major business changes, which of the following is likely to be closest to the number of houses he painted in 2005?
   a. 25
   b. 31
   c. 22
   d. 45

23. Which of the following values is *not* equal to 12(45 – 8)?
   a. 540 – 96
   b. 12 x 45 – 12 x 8
   c. (-8 + 45) 12
   d. 45 (12 – 8)

24. Which of the following fractions is equal to 4/5?
   a. 8/15
   b. 16/25
   c. 12/15
   d. 28/40

25. A house is 25 feet tall and a ladder is set up 35 feet away from the side of the house. Approximately how long is the ladder from the ground to the roof of the house?
   a. 43 ft
   b. 25 ft
   c. 50 ft
   d. 62 ft

26. Derek received 6 job offers from the 15 interviews he did last month. Which ratio best describes the relationship between the number of jobs he was not offered and the number of jobs for which he interviewed?
   a. 6/15
   b. 15/6
   c. 3/5
   d. 2/3

Use the following table to answer questions 27 – 29.

Mrs. McConnell's Classroom	
Eye Color	**Number of Students**
Brown	14
Blue	9
Hazel	5
Green	2

27. What percentage of students in Mrs. McConnell's classroom has either hazel eyes or green eyes?
   a. 23%
   b. 30%
   c. 47%
   d. 77%

28. How many more students have either brown or blue eyes than students who have hazel or green eyes?
   a. 23
   b. 7
   c. 16
   d. 14

29. What is the ratio of students with brown eyes to students with green eyes?
   a. 1:2
   b. 3:1
   c. 1:5
   d. 7:1

30. What is 4 2/9 ÷ 2 2/3?
    a. 11 7/27
    b. 1 7/12
    c. 1 1/12
    d. 2 5/12

31. On a map, the space of ½ of an inch represents 15 miles. If two cities are 4 3/5 inches apart on the map, what is the actual distance between the two cities?
    a. 138 miles
    b. 39 miles
    c. 23 miles
    d. 125 miles

32. If Louis travels on his bike at an average rate of 20 mph, how long will it take him to travel 240 miles?
    a. 48 hours
    b. 12 hours
    c. 20 hours
    d. 8 hours

33. Maria paid $28.00 for a jacket that was discounted by 30%. What was the original price of the jacket?
    a. $36.00
    b. $47.60
    c. $40.00
    d. $42.50

34. A soda company is testing a new sized can to put on the market. The new can is 6 inches in diameter and 12 inches in height. What is the volume of the can in cubic inches?
    a. 339
    b. 113
    c. 432
    d. 226

35. What is the product of 41.20 and 10.5?
    a. 43.260
    b. 4.326
    c. 43,260
    d. 432.60

36. A garden has a perimeter of 600 yards. If the length of the garden is 250 yards, what is the garden's width?
    a. 25
    b. 50
    c. 175
    d. 350

37. Which of the following values is greatest?
    a. -4 minus 10
    b. -25 – (-30)
    c. 4(-20)
    d. -2(-10)

38. A farmer set up a rain gauge in his field and recorded the following daily precipitation amounts over the course of a week: 0.45 inches, 0.0 inches, 0.75 inches, 1.20 inches, 1.1 inches, 0.2 inches, and 0.0 inches. What was the average precipitation over that week?
    a. 0.74 in
    b. 1.05 in
    c. 0.53 in
    d. 3.70 in

39. 25% of what number is 80?
    a. 200
    b. 320
    c. 160
    d. 135

40. Tony has the following number of T-shirts in his closet:
    White - 5
    Black - 2
    Blue - 1
    Yellow - 3
If Tony's electricity goes out, how many T-shirts would he have to pull out of his closet to make sure he has a yellow T-shirt?
    a. 4
    b. 8
    c. 9
    d. 11

41. While at the airport, Adrienne shops for perfume because the product is duty-free, meaning there is no sales tax. If she makes a purchase of $55.00 and the sales tax in that city is 7%, how much money has she saved?
    a. $3.85
    b. $0.38
    c. $7.85
    d. $4.65

42. Enrique is a full-time employee who earns $12.00 per hour. If he works overtime, he receives time-and-a-half (where each hour worked over 40 hours is compensated at 1.5 times the regular rate). If Enrique works 45 hours, how much money will he earn?
    a. $540
    b. $570
    c. $510
    d. $600

43. What is 825.4589 rounded to the nearest tenths place?
    a. 825.46
    b. 825.5
    c. 825.4
    d. 825

44. How many feet are in 5 1/3 yards?
    a. 15
    b. 1 7/9
    c. 15 1/3
    d. 16

45. At a company's annual picnic luncheon, ¼ of the people bring hamburgers, ½ of the people bring potato chips and 1/6 of the people bring soda. Approximately what percentage of people did not bring hamburgers, potato chips, or soda?
    a. 8%
    b. 40%
    c. 25%
    d. 10%

Science and Technical Reasoning

DIRECTIONS: The science and technical reasoning practice test you are about to take is multiple-choice with only one correct answer per question. Read each test item and circle your answer on the answer sheet below. When you have completed the practice test, you may check your answers with those on the answer key that follows the test.

Answer Sheet

1.   a   b   c   d
2.   a   b   c   d
3.   a   b   c   d
4.   a   b   c   d
5.   a   b   c   d
6.   a   b   c   d
7.   a   b   c   d
8.   a   b   c   d
9.   a   b   c   d
10. a   b   c   d
11. a   b   c   d
12. a   b   c   d
13. a   b   c   d
14. a   b   c   d
15. a   b   c   d
16. a   b   c   d
17. a   b   c   d
18. a   b   c   d
19. a   b   c   d
20. a   b   c   d
21. a   b   c   d
22. a   b   c   d
23. a   b   c   d
24. a   b   c   d
25. a   b   c   d
26. a   b   c   d
27. a   b   c   d
28. a   b   c   d
29. a   b   c   d
30. a   b   c   d

Science and Technical Reasoning Test

1. Which of the following correctly lists the cellular hierarchy from the simplest to the most complex structure?
   a. tissue, cell, organ, organ system, organism
   b. organism, organ system, organ, tissue, cell
   c. organ system, organism, organ, tissue, cell
   d. cell, tissue, organ, organ system, organism

2. If a cell is placed in a hypertonic solution, what will happen to the cell?
   a. It will swell.
   b. It will shrink.
   c. It will stay the same.
   d. It does not affect the cell.

3. What is the longest phase of the cell cycle?
   a. mitosis
   b. cytokinesis
   c. interphase
   d. metaphase

Use the following Punnett Square to answer questions 4 and 5.

B = alleles for brown eyes; g = alleles for green eyes

	B	G
B	BB	Bg
g	Bg	gg

4. Which word describes the allele for green eyes?
   a. dominant
   b. recessive
   c. homozygous
   d. heterozygous

5. What is the possibility that the offspring produced will have brown eyes?
   a. 25%
   b. 50%
   c. 75%
   d. 100%

6. What are groups of cells that perform the same function called?
   a. tissues
   b. plastids
   c. organs
   d. molecules

7. When does the nuclear division of somatic cells take place during cellular reproduction?
   a. meiosis
   b. cytokinesis
   c. interphase
   d. mitosis

8. Which group of major parts and organs make up the immune system?
   a. lymphatic system, spleen, tonsils, thymus, and bone marrow
   b. brain, spinal cord, and nerve cells
   c. heart, veins, arteries, and capillaries
   d. nose, trachea, bronchial tubes, lungs, alveolus, and diaphragm

9. The rate of a chemical reaction depends on all of the following except
   a. temperature.
   b. surface area.
   c. presence of catalysts.
   d. amount of mass lost.

10. Which of the answer choices provided best defines the following statement?
    For a given mass and constant temperature, an inverse relationship exists between the volume and pressure of a gas?
    a. Ideal Gas Law
    b. Boyle's Law
    c. Charles' Law
    d. Stefan-Boltzmann Law

11. Which of the following statement correctly compares prokaryotic and eukaryotic cells?
    a. Prokaryotic cells have a true nucleus, eukaryotic cells do not.
    b. Both prokaryotic and eukaryotic cells have a membrane.
    c. Prokaryotic cells do not contain organelles, eukaryotic cells do.
    d. Prokaryotic cells are more complex than eukaryotic cells.

12. What is the role of ribosomes?
    a. make proteins
    b. waste removal
    c. transport
    d. storage

13. Which of the following is an example of a tissue?
    a. chloroplast
    b. liver
    c. mammal
    d. hamstring

14. The adrenal glands are part of the
    a. immune system.
    b. endocrine system.
    c. emphatic system.
    d. respiratory system.

15. Which of the following is exchanged between two or more atoms that undergo ionic bonding?
    a. neutrons
    b. transitory electrons
    c. valence electrons
    d. electrical charges

16. Which of the following statements is *not* true of most metals?
    a. They are good conductors of heat.
    b. They are gases at room temperature.
    c. They are ductile.
    d. They make up the majority of elements on the periodic table.

17. What is most likely the pH of a solution containing many hydroxide ions (OH^-) and few hydrogen ions (H^+)?
    a. 2
    b. 6
    c. 7
    d. 9

18. Which of the following cannot be found on the periodic table?
    a. bromine
    b. magnesium oxide
    c. phosphorous
    d. chlorine

19. Nora makes soup by adding some spices to a pot of boiling water and stirring the spices until completely dissolved. Next, she adds several chopped vegetables. What is the solute in her mixture?
    a. water
    b. vegetables
    c. spices
    d. heat

20. A cyclist is riding over a hill. At what point is his potential energy greatest?
    a. at the base of the hill
    b. halfway up the hill
    c. at the very top of the hill
    d. on the way down the hill

21. Which of the following correctly describes the trait Ll, if "L" represents tallness and "l" represents shortness?
    a. heterozygous genotype and tall phenotype
    b. heterozygous phenotype and tall genotype
    c. homozygous genotype and short phenotype
    d. homozygous phenotype and short genotype

22. Which of the following waves is a type of electromagnetic wave?
    a. ocean wave
    b. sound wave
    c. transverse wave
    d. gamma wave

23. Hemoglobin transports oxygen from the lungs to the rest of the body, making oxygen available for cell use. What is hemoglobin?
    a. an enzyme
    b. a protein
    c. a lipid
    d. an acid

24. Which of the following is an example of a non-communicable disease?
    a. influenza
    b. tuberculosis
    c. arthritis
    d. measles

25. Which of the following statements describes the function of smooth muscle tissue?
    a. It contracts to force air into and out of the lungs.
    b. It contracts to force air into and out of the stomach.
    c. It contracts to support the spinal column.
    d. It contracts to assist the stomach in the mechanical breakdown of food.

26. What law describes the electric force between two charged particles?
    a. Ohm's law
    b. Coulomb's law
    c. The Doppler effect
    d. Kirchhoff's current law

27. Which of the following is not a product of respiration?
    a. carbon dioxide
    b. water
    c. glucose
    d. ATP

28. Which of the following compose the central nervous system?
    a. the brain and spinal cord
    b. the brain and heart
    c. the heart and lungs
    d. all the muscles in the body

29. What process transfers thermal energy through matter directly from particle to particle?
    a. convection
    b. radiation
    c. conduction
    d. insulation

30. Which state of matter contains the least amount of kinetic energy?
    a. solid
    b. liquid
    c. gas
    d. plasma

English and Language Usage

DIRECTIONS: The English and language usage practice test you are about to take is multiple-choice with only one correct answer per question. Read each test item and circle your answer on the answer sheet below. When you have completed the practice test, you may check your answers with those answers on the answer key that follows the test.

Answer Sheet

1.	a	b	c	d		29.	a	b	c	d
2.	a	b	c	d		30.	a	b	c	d
3.	a	b	c	d		31.	a	b	c	d
4.	a	b	c	d		32.	a	b	c	d
5.	a	b	c	d		33.	a	b	c	d
6.	a	b	c	d		34.	a	b	c	d
7.	a	b	c	d		35.	a	b	c	d
8.	a	b	c	d		36.	a	b	c	d
9.	a	b	c	d		37.	a	b	c	d
10.	a	b	c	d		38.	a	b	c	d
11.	a	b	c	d		39.	a	b	c	d
12.	a	b	c	d		40.	a	b	c	d
13.	a	b	c	d		41.	a	b	c	d
14.	a	b	c	d		42.	a	b	c	d
15.	a	b	c	d		43.	a	b	c	d
16.	a	b	c	d		44.	a	b	c	d
17.	a	b	c	d		45.	a	b	c	d
18.	a	b	c	d		46.	a	b	c	d
19.	a	b	c	d		47.	a	b	c	d
20.	a	b	c	d		48.	a	b	c	d
21.	a	b	c	d		49.	a	b	c	d
22.	a	b	c	d		50.	a	b	c	d
23.	a	b	c	d		51.	a	b	c	d
24.	a	b	c	d		52.	a	b	c	d
25.	a	b	c	d		53.	a	b	c	d
26.	a	b	c	d		54.	a	b	c	d
27.	a	b	c	d		55.	a	b	c	d
28.	a	b	c	d						

English and Language Usage Test

Questions 1-30 pertain to the following passage. Read the passage and correct the underlined words or phrases.

Danny and Carla (1) <u>were being married</u> for two years. For (2) <u>there</u> honeymoon, they (3) <u>had</u> gone to the Grand Cayman Island for a nice, relaxing vacation at a luxury beach resort. But their honeymoon turned out to be anything but relaxing.

When (4) <u>they were arriving</u> at the airport, they hailed a taxi. The taxi driver strapped the suitcases to the top of the car and sped off towards the resort. Along the way, the taxi driver swerved (5) <u>to avoid hit</u> a cat on the road. This caused (6) <u>Carla'</u> suitcase to fly off the car and crash in the road. Her clothes, shoes, and personal items (7) <u>had flown</u> everywhere. She yelled (8) <u>anger</u> at the driver to stop immediately. Danny and Carla rushed out of the cab to gather her belongings. Once they collected everything they (9) <u>can find</u>, they started again for the resort. When they finally arrived, the driver charged them for the time spent collecting the things on the road. Irate, Danny made sure not to tip him.

Exhausted, Danny and Carla checked into their room. When they got to the room, they noticed they did not have a beachfront view as they (10) <u>had been promised</u>. They were also in a smoking room even though they had requested a non-smoking room. Danny asked to switch rooms, but the concierge (11) <u>apollageticaly</u> replied that they were booked for the rest of the week. "(12) <u>Its</u> a popular week for tourists, sir," she replied. Nothing (13) <u>could be done</u>. Danny, (14) <u>that</u> was trying to stay positive, told Carla not to worry. As long as they kept the windows open, the smell of cigarettes would not be (15) <u>to</u> much of a bother.

The next day, they (16) <u>waked up</u> early to fish and then go to the beach. They walked (17) <u>at the beach</u> and found a small table, two chairs, and a large umbrella. Then, they rented a boat to fish. Carla caught only one fish, but Danny (18) <u>catched several fishes</u>. When they got back, they took a nap on the beach. They finally felt peaceful. A few minutes later, a large family with six kids took a space right next to them. The kids were loud. Some of the kids were arguing, while some ran around squealing in delight. Danny and Carla were unable to sleep, so Danny suggested they (19) <u>went for a walk</u> together. Not paying attention to where they were walking, Carla suddenly jumped up and screamed in agony. She had stepped on a jellyfish and (20) <u>had got</u> stung. She was in pain and couldn't walk, so Danny (21) <u>had carried</u> her all the way back to the room.

Back (22) <u>into the room,</u> Danny (23) <u>realizing they had left</u> their things at the beach. Just as he was about to get them, it started to (24) <u>poor</u>. Danny hoped the umbrella would keep their things dry, but the wind (25) <u>was knocked</u> the umbrella over and everything (26) <u>were soaked</u>. Their books, phones, and wallet (27) <u>was ruinned</u>. To make matters worse, the rain didn't stop. Two days (28) <u>went by</u>. They had to stay in their smelly room, Carla was still in pain, and Danny was in a bad mood. Needless to say, they (29) <u>gone</u> home early. They thought they might be able to get their money back from the travel agent, but that was also (30) <u>unsuccessfull</u>.

Questions: Passage I

1.
    a. no change
    b. were been married
    c. have been married
    d. were married

2.
    a. no change
    b. their
    c. they're
    d. theyre

3.
    a. no change
    b. had went
    c. gone
    d. went

4.
    a. no change
    b. they were arrived
    c. they arrived
    d. they are arriving

5.
    a. no change
    b. to avoid hitting
    c. to avoid hiting
    d. to avoid hitted

6.
    a. no change
    b. Carlas
    c. Carlas'
    d. Carla's

7.
    a. no change
    b. flyed
    c. flew
    d. flown

8.
    a. no change
    b. in an angry way
    c. angrily
    d. angrier

9.
    a. no change
    b. can found
    c. could find
    d. could found

10.
      a. no change
      b. were being promised
      c. are promised
      d. promised

11.
      a. no change
      b. apologetically
      c. apollogetically
      d. apollagetically

12.
      a. no change
      b. It
      c. It's
      d. It was

13.
      a. no change
      b. could have done
      c. could done
      d. could been done

14.
      a. no change
      b. whose
      c. who
      d. which

15.
      a. no change
      b. two
      c. too
      d. soo

16.
      a. no change
      b. woken up
      c. woked up
      d. woke up

17.
      a. no change
      b. to the beach
      c. in the beach
      d. for the beach

18.
      a. no change
      b. catched several fish
      c. caught several fish
      d. caught several fishes

19.
      a. no change
      b. go for a walk
      c. going for a walk
      d. had gone for a walk

20.
    a. no change
    b. had get
    c. got
    d. gotten
21.
    a. no change
    b. was carried
    c. was carrying
    d. carried
22.
    a. no change
    b. in the room
    c. for the room
    d. on the room
23.
    a. no change
    b. had realized they had left
    c. realized they had left
    d. realizing they were leaving
24.
    a. no change
    b. pour
    c. porre
    d. pore
25.
    a. no change
    b. was knock
    c. knocking
    d. had knocked
26.
    a. no change
    b. was soaked
    c. were soaking
    d. was soak
27.
    a. no change
    b. was ruined
    c. were ruined
    d. were ruinned
28.
    a. no change
    b. gone by
    c. went
    d. gone past
29.
    a. no change
    b. had gone
    c. went
    d. will be going

30.
      a. no change
      b. unsuccessful
      c. unsucesful
      d. unsuccesful

Answer the following items.

31. Writing, doing yoga, and _____ were her favorite activities.
      a. playing volleyball
      b. doing volleyball
      c. making volleyball
      d. volleyballing

32. Which sentence is written correctly?
      a. The student, who was caught cheating, was given detention.
      b. The student who was caught cheating was given detention.
      c. The student who was caught cheating, was given detention.
      d. The student; who was caught cheating; was given detention.

33. Which sentence is written most clearly?
      a. His neighbor's dog was walked for an allowance by the boy.
      b. The boy walked his neighbor's dog for an allowance.
      c. For an allowance, the boy walked the dog of his neighbor's.
      d. The dog of his neighbor's was walked by the boy for an allowance.

34. Every kid in the neighborhood has _____ own bicycle.
      a. its
      b. their
      c. our
      d. her

Read the following weather forecast and answer questions 35 – 39.

The weather will remain capricious over the next few days, with intermittent rain possible during the forecast period. Temperatures will generally be above the average high of 75° F, but expect some locations to climb into the low 80s. Tonight's lows will be mild around 55° F, with the outlying areas staying relatively cooler. Winds in the morning should be constant at 7 mph but will increase by up to three times by the afternoon as a cold front encroaches.

35. What does <u>capricious</u> mean?
      a. steady
      b. unpredictable
      c. pleasant
      d. violent

36. What is the normal high temperature for this time of year?
    a. low 80s
    b. 75° – 80° F
    c. 75° F
    d. 65° F

37. What does <u>intermittent</u> mean?
    a. occasional
    b. intense
    c. frequent
    d. bursts

38. According to the forecast, what will the wind speed be around 4:00 that   afternoon?
    a. 7 mph
    b. 10 mph
    c. 14 mph
    d. 21 mph

39. Which of the following words could replace the word <u>encroaches</u> in the passage?
    a. invades
    b. approaches
    c. retreats
    d. influences

Read the paragraph below to answer questions 40 – 43.

Here are the safety rules for novice scuba divers. These rules are essential to ensure a safe and fun experience. Most importantly, listen to your guide's instructions. The maximum depth of any dive is 100 feet. Make a safety stop for a few minutes at about fifteen feet. Always dive with a partner. If you lose your partner or group you may search for them, but only for a minute. If you cannot find them, then resurface. Do not touch or disturb any fauna or flora, as you may get stung or bitten. Also, do not collect anything from the water in order to preserve the health of the ecosystem and not disturb marine life. Only garbage may be removed. In the event that you are caught in a current, stay calm and relax. It is better to float to the surface and signal for help than to fight against the current. Lastly, stay aware of any changing conditions during the dive. Make sure you finish your dive with at least 40 bars of oxygen left in your tank. Consider that if conditions worsen or become unpredictable, it may be necessary to end the dive prematurely.

40. What should a diver do if separated from the group?
    a. Immediately signal for help.
    b. Look for them until they are found.
    c. Look for them for a short period then return to the surface.
    d. Stay in the same place for a long period and wait for them to find you.

41. At what depth should a diver make a safety stop?
    a. 15 feet below the surface
    b. 15 feet above the ocean floor
    c. 85 feet below the surface
    d. a few feet below the surface

42. If the diver sees a school of fish, which of the following would the diver be allowed to do?
    a. touch the fish to assess the texture of its skin
    b. catch the fish to cook for dinner
    c. observe the fish from a distance
    d. poke the fish with a long pole to study its behavior

43. Why might it be important to finish a dive with a minimum of 40 bars of oxygen in the tank?
    a. to avoid running out of oxygen and have extra in case of emergency
    b. to have enough oxygen saved with which to begin the next dive
    c. to have enough oxygen in case you need to swim against a current
    d. it is impossible to know how much oxygen is needed to reach the surface and get back to the boat

Fill in the blanks for questions 44 through 48.

44. Maria thinks it is unfair that she has to _____ with her younger brother's whining all the time.
    a. put up
    b. put down
    c. put in
    d. put off

45. Enrique will _____ harder as the date of the test draws nearer.
    a. studying
    b. have studied
    c. studyed
    d. study

46. Suzanna replied _____ to her sister's plea to help her with her finances.
    a. sympathelly
    b. sympathetically
    c. sympathetilly
    d. sympathetic

47. A team of scientists _____ studying a new species of frog never found before.
    a. is
    b. are
    c. were
    d. have

48. Everyone we invited to the party _____, so it was a huge success!
    a. shown up
    b. showed up
    c. showed upped
    d. shows up

Identify the misspelled word in the sentences below.

49. Rudy beleives you should focus on your children more than on your marriage,   due to the complexities of young minds.
    a. beleives
    b. focus
    c. complexities
    d. marriage

50. Buying prescents for others is not the most authentic way to develop new friendships.
    a. buying
    b. prescents
    c. authentic
    d. friendships

51. Raymond feels children misbehave too much, that parents have lost their athourity, and that they need to emphasize discipline more.
    a. misbehave
    b. emphasize
    c. discipline
    d. athourity

52. Larry travelled to India to participate in a pilgrimage across the Indian countryside hoping to relinquish all stress and achieve peace.
    a. travelled
    b. pilgrimage
    c. relinquish
    d. achieve

Choose the meaning of the underlined words in the sentences below.

53. The group hiked along a <u>precipitous</u> slope that many found unnerving.
    a. ugged
    b. dangerous
    c. steep
    d. wet

54. Saline is taking a philosophy class but finds most of the readings to be very <u>obscure</u>, so she has not benefited much from them.
    a. opinionated
    b. unclear
    c. offensive
    d. benign

55. As a young boy, Dorian was <u>remiss</u> about his homework and failed to get good grades in school.
    a. timely
    b. diligent
    c. negligent
    d. meticulous

Answer Key

	Reading	Mathematics	Science	English
1	B	B	D	C
2	A	C	B	B
3	D	D	C	D
4	C	A	B	C
5	A	B	C	B
6	D	A	A	D
7	B	B	D	C
8	D	D	A	C
9	C	C	D	C
10	B	B	B	A
11	A	C	C	B
12	C	D	A	C
13	C	B	A	A
14	B	C	B	C
15	D	A	C	C
16	C	B	B	D
17	B	A	D	B
18	B	B	B	C
19	A	D	C	B
20	D	B	C	C
21	A	A	A	D
22	C	B	D	B
23	B	D	B	C
24	C	C	C	B
25	B	A	D	D
26	A	C	B	B
27	D	A	C	C
28	C	C	A	A
29	C	D	C	C
30	A	B	A	B
31	D	A		A
32	B	B		B
33	D	C		B
34	A	A		D
35	B	D		B
36	D	B		C
37	C	D		A
38	A	C		D
39	D	B		B
40	C	C		C
41		A		A
42		B		C
43		B		A

	Reading	Mathematics	Science	English
44		D		A
45		A		D
46				B
47				A
48				B
49				A
50				B
51				D
52				A
53				C
54				B
55				C

Reading Answer Explanations

1. B
Explanation: The passage was written to analyze the works by Chang-Rae Lee and the themes presented in his most famous novels.

2. A
Explanation: The author of this passage uses the first line of the novel to provide an example of one of the themes of the novel.

3. D
Explanation: Espionage is part of the plot of the novel <u>Native Speaker</u>, but it is not a theme that recurs in Lee's works.

4. C
Explanation: The passage states that Lee's interests in cultural identity and race emerge from his own experiences with these issues as a young immigrant to America.

5. A
Explanation: The tone of the last paragraph suggests concern over the preservation of cultural identities in an increasingly mixed and expanding world.

6. D
Explanation: The passage indicates that the formula increases or boosts the absorption of minerals in the body.

7. B
Explanation: The directions say to mix equal parts of all the herbs listed.

8. D
Explanation: The dosage indicates not to exceed four tablespoons in a 24-hour period, so the patient should take it no more than every six hours.

9. C
Explanation: All methods are used in the cooking process except for whisking.

10. B
Explanation: Albany received 0.55 inches of rain, while Bunbury received only 0.20 in. 0.55 − 0.20 = 0.35 inches.

11. A
Explanation: Looking at the fifth day of the month, you get: 0.90 + 1.01 + 0.50 = 2.41 ÷ 3 = 0.80.

12. C
Explanation: Flooding would be of greatest concern on the day that received the most rain in each location, the 6th.

13. C
Explanation: By summing the total amount of precipitation received over the week, Bunbury received less than Albany and Coral Bay.

14. B
Explanation: By comparing the differences between Albany and Coral Bay, Coral Bay is typically a little wetter on average than Albany.

15. D
Explanation: In one month, 2,000 m or 2 km of tunnel could be built with 2 machines. 2 km/1 month = 50 km/x; 2x = 50; x = 25 months, or just over 2 years.

16. C
Explanation: It takes 3 hrs and 10 mins to travel from London to Brussels, so with the one hour time change, a person on the 8:35 a.m. train would arrive in Brussels at 12:45 p.m., local time.

17. B
Explanation: The passage does not say anything about concerns over how long the construction would take to complete.

18. B
Explanation: Vehement most closely means the same thing as intense.

19. A
Explanation: Diatribe most closely means the same thing as criticism.

20. D
Explanation: Cogitate most closely means the same thing as deliberate.

21. A
Explanation: Invidious most closely means the same thing as offensive.

22. C
Explanation: Hyperbole most closely means the same thing as exaggeration.

23. B
Explanation: Innocuous most closely means the same thing as innocent.

24. C
Explanation: The professor argues that after a fire, small, woody material is left on the tops of trees where a fire cannot reach. Therefore, the material is unavailable as fuel for future fires.

25. B
Explanation: Since the plot that was salvage logged (Plot A) burned with greater severity than the unmanaged plot (Plot B), the study supports the professor's view that salvage logging increases the risk and severity of fire.

26. A
Explanation: The forest manager feels that by removing dead or dying material through salvage logging, less fuel is available for future fires.

27. D
Explanation: The professor states the opposite of answer choice D and says that larger trees found in old growth forests are more resistant to fire than small, younger trees.

28. C
Explanation: A study looking at the regeneration of seedlings in both logged and unmanaged forests would help to clarify and/or validate both arguments, since both the manager and the professor discuss the importance of seedling growth following a fire.

29. C
Explanation: The passage states that he was given this title since he was the first to explain how organisms change over time.

30. A
Explanation: The tone and purpose of this passage is to inform the reader.

31. D
Explanation: The passage explains that finches with longer, sharper beaks were able to reach insects more easily than finches with shorter beaks, giving them an advantage over the other finches on the island.

32. B
Explanation: The island finches were different from the mainland finches, so their geographical separation over time increased the diversity of finches.

33. D
Explanation: The passage states that the island finches differed from the mainland finches by the shape of their beaks and in their diet.

34. A
Explanation: While the other answer choices may be valid reasons, the passage clearly states that residents hope to reduce emissions associated with bottling and transporting the water.

35. B
Explanation: The passage states that residents want to lessen the impact raising livestock has on the environment, namely to reduce the emissions from the livestock industry.

36. D
Explanation: There is a majority in favor of the ban, with 400 people for it and only 2 people against it.

37. C
Explanation: The Eagle Eye Trail is the only trail that does not connect to one of the other trails.

38. A

Explanation: The Beaverton Falls trail is an easy trail and says that it is suitable for people of all ages. It also offers picnic areas. The other trails listed are moderate to hard and do not offer areas to picnic.

39. D

Explanation: According to the table, the Toulanne Trail offers boat rentals as early as May; whereas, the Silver Bullet Trail does not allow fishing until July.

40. C

Explanation: The total distance they will hike is 2.6 miles + 9.5 miles =12.1 miles. If they hike 3 miles per hour, it will take them 12.1/3 = 4.03 hours to hike 12.1 miles.

Mathematics Answer Explanations

1. B

Explanation: The relationship can be expressed as: $15/10 = 45/x$; $15x = 450$; $x = 30$.

2. C

Explanation: The total amount of the bill is: $3.70/x = 8/100$; $370 = 8x$; $x = \$46.25$.

3. D

Explanation: First set the relationship up and solve for the number of packs: $x/2=5/packs$; $x(packs) = 10$; $packs = 10/x$.

4. A

Explanation: The correct expression is: $J = 1/2K + 5$.

5. B

Explanation: If $E + B = 225$, and $E = 2B + 5$, then $225 – B = 2B + 5$. Solving for B, $3B = 220$ and $B = 73.3$. $225 – 73.3 = 151.7$.

6. A

Explanation: Plugging in x and y, you get $(4(3) – 4) + (-10 + 4)$, which is $8 + (-6)$, or $8 – 6 = 2$.

7. B

Explanation: The average rate of cooling is: $(86º - 38º) / 9$ hrs; $48º / 9 = 5.33º$ F per hour.

8. D

Explanation: Calculate the weighted average of the 3 tests: $(80+75+92) / 3 = 82.3$; Calculate the average of the 2 oral quizzes: $(22/25) \times 100 = 88$ and $(19/25) \times 100 = 76$, so $(88 + 76)/2 = 82$. Multiply each grade by their weight, and then add them all up to determine the final grade: $(82 \times .45) + (88 \times .25) + (91 \times .15) + (82 \times .15) = 85$.

9. C

- 46 -

Explanation: Calculate the average price as [(3.5 x 2) + (0.3 x 5) + (1.25 x 3) + (0.45 x 6)] / (2 + 5 + 3 + 6) = 0.93.

10. B
Explanation: 68% = 68/100. To express as a fraction, move the decimal two places to the left, .68.

11. C
Explanation: 2 1/7 x 3 2/3 = 15/7 x 11/3 = 165/21 = 7 18/21 = 7 6/7.

12. D
Explanation: Remember the order of operations: (27 ÷ 9) = 3 and ($\sqrt{25}$ x 2) = 10; 3 x 10 = 30.

13. B
Explanation: Double the number that is added to the previous number. So, 4+2=6, 6+4=10, 10+8=18, 18+16=34, and 34+32=66.

14. C
Explanation: An improper fraction is one whose numerator is greater than the denominator.

15. A
Explanation: 1 kilometer is equal to 100,000 centimeters. 250/10000 = .0025.

16. B
Explanation: 144 x 0.40 = 57.6 + 144 = 201.6 and 168 x 0.40 = 67.2 + 168 = 235.2; then, convert to feet: 201.6/12 = 16.8 ft and 235.2/12 = 19.6 ft.

17. A
Explanation: $(x^2)^3 = x^{(2 \times 3)} = x^6$; $(y^2)^5 = y^{(2 \times 5)} = y^{10}$; $(y^4)^3 = y^{(4 \times 3)} = y^{12}$; $y^{10} \cdot y^{12} = y^{(10+12)} = y^{22}$.

18. B
Explanation: $(x^2)^5 y^6 z^2 / x^4 (y^3)^4 z^2 = x^{(2 \times 5)} - x^4 = x^{10} - x^4 = x^6$; $y^6 - y^{(3 \times 4)} = y^6 - y^{12} = y^{-6}$; $z^2 - z^2 = z^0$ or 0; so the answer is: $x^6 y^{-6}$.

19. D
Explanation: 1 gallon = 128 ounces, so 8 x 128 = 1,024 ounces for 8 gallons. ½ = 64 gallons, and ¼ = 32 gallons, so 64 + 32 = 96 ounces to fill the ¾ gallons; the total ounces required is 1,024 + 96 = 1,120 ounces.

20. B
Explanation: If mangoes are represented by x and coconuts are represented by y, then:
    x + y = 10, and 2x + 4y = 30
    2(10-y) + 4y = 30
    20 – 2y + 4y = 30
    2y = 10
    y = 5 and x = 5, or 5 of each type of fruit

21. A
Explanation: The average number of houses painted is: 5 + 9 + 15 + 20 + 25 / 5 = 14.8 or 15.

22. B
Explanation: Given the increasing trend, the data can be extrapolated from 25 to about 31, the closest possible answer.

23. D
Explanation: 12(45 − 8) = 540 − 96 = 444, but 45(12 − 8) = 540 − 360 = 180.

24. C
Explanation: The least common multiple of the fraction 12/15 is 3, lending 4/5.

25. A
Explanation: Using the Pythagorean theorem: $25^2 + 35^2 = c^2$. $625 + 1225 = c^2$. c = sqrt 1850 = 43.01.

26. C
Explanation: The number of jobs he did not get is 15 − 6 = 9. The ratio is 9:15 or 3:5.

27. A
Explanation: Total # of students = 14 + 9 + 5 + 2 = 30. 5 + 2 = 7. 7/30 = X/100. 700 = 30X. X = 23.3.

28. C
Explanation: 14 + 9 = 23 and 5 + 2 = 7. 23 − 7 = 16.

29. D
Explanation: Brown eyes = 14 and Green eyes = 2. So, the ratio is 14:2 or 7:1.

30. B
Explanation: 4 2/9 = 38/9 and 2 2/3 = 8/3. 38/9 ÷ 8/3 = 38/9 x 3/8. 114/72 = 57/36 = 19/12 = 1 7/12.

31. A
Explanation: ½ / 15 = 4 3/5 / X; ½ X = 15 x 23/5. ½ X = 69. X = 69 x 2 = 138.

32. B
Explanation: 20/1 = 240/X. 20X = 240. X = 240/20 = 12 hours.

33. C
Explanation: If X represents the original price of the jacket and Y represents the discounted amount, then 0.30X = Y and X − Y = 28; X − 0.30X = 28; 0.70X = 28; X = 28/.70 = 40.

34. A
Explanation: $V = \pi r^2 h$. V = 3.14 x (3^2) x 12. 3.14 x 9 x 12 = 339.12.

35. D
Explanation: The decimals are counted as 3 spaces from the right, so 41.20 x 10.5 = 432.600.

36. B
Explanation: The equation for perimeter (P) = 2L + 2W. So, 600 = 2(250) + 2W. Solve for W: 600 − 500 = 2W. 100 = 2W. W = 50.

37. D
Explanation: Multiplying a negative number by another negative number yields a positive number, in this case -2 x -10 = +20, which is the largest answer choice.

38. C
Explanation: (0.45 + 0.0 + 0.75 + 1.20 + 1.1 + 0.2 + 0.0) / 7 = 0.53.

39. B
Explanation: (0.25)X = 80. X = 80/0.25. X = 320.

40. C
Explanation: He would have to pull out at least 9 (5 + 2 + 1 + 1) to make sure he has a yellow one.

41. A
Explanation: 55 x 7/100 = 55 x .07 = 3.85.

42. B
Explanation: He gets paid $12.00/hr for the first 40 hrs: 12 x 40 = $480. For time-and-a-half: 5 x 1.5 = 7.5. 7.5 x 12 = $90. So, 480 + 90 = $570.

43. B
Explanation: The tenths place is the first place to the right of the decimal. 825.4589 should be rounded up to 825.5.

44. D
Explanation: 1 yard = 3 feet. (5 1/3 yards / X) x (3 feet/1 yard) = 16/3 x 3 = 48/3. X = 16.

45. A
Explanation: ¼ + ½ + 1/6 = 3/12 + 6/12 + 2/12 = 11/12. 12/12 – 11/12 = 1/12. 1/12 = .083 = 8%.

Science Answer Explanations

1. D
Explanation: The cellular hierarchy starts with the cell, the simplest structure, and progresses to organisms, the most complex structures.

2. B
Explanation: A hypertonic solution is a solution with a higher particle concentration than in the cell, and consequently lower water content than in the cell. Water moves from the cell to the solution, causing the cell to experience water loss and shrink.

3. C
Explanation: Interphase is the period when the DNA is replicated (or when the chromosomes are replicated) and is the longest part of the cell cycle.

4. B

Explanation: Recessive alleles are represented by lower case letters, while dominant alleles are represented by upper case letters,

5. C
Explanation: Dominant genes are always expressed when both alleles are dominant (BB) or when one is dominant and one is recessive (Bg). In this case, ¾ or 75% will have brown eyes.

6. A
Explanation: Groups of cells that perform the same function are called tissues.

7. D
Explanation: The nuclear division of somatic cells takes place during mitosis.

8. A
Explanation: The immune system consists of the lymphatic system, spleen, tonsils, thymus and bone marrow.

9. D
Explanation: The rate at which a chemical reaction occurs does not depend on the amount of mass lost, since the law of conservation of mass (or matter) states that in a chemical reaction there is no loss of mass.

10. B
Explanation: Boyle's law states that for a constant mass and temperature, pressure and volume are related inversely to one another: PV = c, where c = constant.

11. C
Explanation: Prokaryotic cells are simpler cells that do not have membrane-bound organelles, whereas eukaryotic cells have several membrane-bound organelles.

12. A
Explanation: A ribosome is a structure of eukaryotic cells that makes proteins.

13. A
Explanation: A chloroplast is an example of a tissue. A liver is an organ, a mammal is a type of organism, and a hamstring is a muscle.

14. B
Explanation: The adrenal glands are part of the endocrine system. They sit on the kidneys and produce hormones that regulate salt and water balance and influence blood pressure and heart rate.

15. C
Explanation: An ionic bond forms when one atom donates an electron from its outer shell, called a valence electron, to another atom to form two oppositely charged atoms.

16. B
Explanation: Metals are usually solids at room temperature, while nonmetals are usually gases at room temperature.

17. D

Explanation: A solution that contains more hydroxide ions than hydrogen ions is a base, and bases have a pH greater than 7, so the only possible answer is D, 9.

18. B

Explanation: Magnesium oxide cannot be found on the periodic table because it is a compound of two elements.

19. C

Explanation: A solute is a substance that is dissolved in another substance. In this case, the solute is the spices.

20. C

Explanation: Potential energy is stored energy. At the top of the hill, the cyclist has the greatest amount of potential energy (and the least amount of kinetic energy) because his motion is decreased and he has the potential of motion in any direction.

21. A

Explanation: The trait Ll describes the genotype of the person or the traits for the genes they carry. It is heterozygous because it contains a dominant gene and a recessive gene. Tallness is the phenotype of the person or the physical expression of the genes they carry, because L for tallness is the dominant gene.

22. D

Explanation: Gamma waves are the smallest wavelengths of the electromagnetic spectrum.

23. B

Explanation: Hemoglobin is a type of protein found in the red blood cells of all mammals.

24. C

Explanation: Arthritis is a type of non-communicable disease because it is not passed from person to person.

25. D

Explanation: Smooth muscle tissue involuntarily contracts to assist the digestive tract by moving the stomach and helping with the breakdown of food.

26. B

Explanation: Coulomb's law describes the electric force between two charged particles. It states that like charges repel and opposite charges attract, and the greater their distance, the less force they will exert on each other.

27. C

Explanation: In respiration, food is used to produce energy as glucose and oxygen that react to produce carbon dioxide, water and ATP.

28. A

Explanation: The central nervous system is the main control center for the human body and is composed of the brain and spinal cord.

29. C
Explanation: Conduction is the transfer of thermal energy between two substances that come into contact with each other; their particles must collide in order to transfer energy.

30. A
Explanation: Solids contain the least amount of kinetic energy because they are made up of closely packed atoms or molecules that are locked in position and exhibit very little movement. Gases and plasmas exhibit the greatest amount of energy.

English and Language Usage Answer Explanations

1. C
Explanation: The correct verb tense in this sentence is the present perfect because it refers to a state of being that began in the past (they got married) but is not yet finished (they are still married).

2. B
Explanation: The correct word is "their." This word is a plural possessive form of "they," whereas the word "there" refers to a place.

3. D
Explanation: The verb "to go" is irregular. The correct tense here is the past simple, "went," instead of the past perfect, "had gone," because the sentence refers to only one finished past action.

4. C
Explanation: The correct verb tense is the past simple "they arrived" instead of the past continuous "they were arriving."

5. B
Explanation: The correct form should be the infinitive plus an -ing verb. The main verb in the sentence, swerved, tells us the action happened in the past.

6. D
Explanation: Carla is a noun that does not end in "s," so the possessive is formed by adding an apostrophe and s, as in "Carla's."

7. C
Explanation: The verb to fly is an irregular verb; the correct form of the past tense is "flew."

8. C
Explanation: This word needs to be in the form of an adverb; the correct spelling is "angrily."

9. C
Explanation: The past tense of the word "can" is "could," so the correct answer is "could find."

- 52 -

10. A

Explanation: This sentence uses the correct verb tense. The past perfect is used because it refers to a past action that happened before another past action.

11. B

Explanation: The correct spelling of the word is "apologetically."

12. C

Explanation: This sentence should use the contraction "it's," meaning "it is." The word "its" refers to the singular possessive.

13. A

Explanation: This sentence correctly uses the word "there."

14. C

Explanation: The correct relative pronoun to use in this relative clause is "who," because the pronoun is referring to a person and is not possessive.

15. C

Explanation: The correct word to use in this sentence is "too," which means "also."

16. D

Explanation: The verb "to wake" is irregular and the past tense is "woke."

17. B

Explanation: The correct prepositional phrase to use here is "to the beach."

18. C

Explanation: The verb "to catch" is irregular and the past tense is "caught." "Fish" is an uncountable noun and the plural form is the same as the singular form, so no "s" is added to make it plural.

19. B

Explanation: The present form of the verb is used here, because the main verb in this phrase is in the past simple, so the second verb should use the infinitive.

20. C

Explanation: The verb should be in the past simple form and not the past perfect, since this action (got stung) happened after the first action in the sentence (had stepped).

21. D

Explanation: The verb tense should be past simple. Past perfect is not needed here because the actions mentioned in the sentence happened one after another in sequence.

22. B

Explanation: The correct prepositional phrase is "in the room."

23. C

Explanation: The correct tense should be past simple (realized) followed by past perfect (had left), because there are two actions and the second action happened before the first action.

24. B
Explanation: This is the wrong word. The correct verb is "pour" which means to rain hard.

25. D
Explanation: The correct verb tense should be past perfect because the action happened before this other action in the past.

26. B
Explanation: The correct verb should be singular, "was soaked," because "everything" is a collective singular noun.

27. C
Explanation: The correct verb is "were," because it refers to three items, not just one. The correct spelling of the verb "ruin" in the past tense is "ruined."

28. A
Explanation: This sentence correctly uses the verb and preposition.

29. C
Explanation: The verb in this sentence, "to go," should use the past simple form, "went." "Gone" is the past participle of "to go."

30. B
Explanation: The correct spelling of the word is "unsuccessful."

31. A
Explanation: Volleyball is a team sport that follows the verb "to play," whereas individual sports like yoga follow the verb "to do."

32. B
Explanation: The term "student" is general, so the relative clause is essential to the meaning of the sentence and should not be separated out by commas.

33. B
Explanation: The second sentence is the clearest, since there are misplaced modifiers and verb confusion in the other sentences.

34. D
Explanation: The word "every" is a singular noun and should be followed by a singular pronoun. In this case, the only singular pronoun is "her."

35. B
Explanation: The word "capricious" means "unpredictable" or "changeable."

36. C
Explanation: The normal temperature is the same as the average temperature, which is 75° F.

37. A
Explanation: The word "intermittent" also means "occasional" or "discontinuous."

38. D
Explanation: The wind speed is expected to be three times as high as in the morning, so 7 x 3 = 21 miles per hour.

39. B
Explanation: Three of the answer choices are synonyms of the word "encroach," but the way it is used in the passage means "to approach."

40. C
Explanation: According to the passage, a diver should spend only a moment looking for others in the group. If the others cannot be found, the diver should resurface.

41. A
Explanation: The passage states that a safety stop should be made fifteen feet down, or below the surface.

42. C
Explanation: Since a diver is not allowed to touch or disturb the fauna in any way, the only activity the diver is allowed to do is observe the fish.

43. A
Explanation: The passage implies that the diver should have enough oxygen left in the tank in case something goes wrong, he or she gets lost, or some other unforeseen complication arises.

44. A
Explanation: The phrasal verb "to put up with" means to have to deal with something or someone.

45. D
Explanation: The future tense is will + the infinitive, in this case "will study."

46. B
Explanation: This should be an adverb, and the correct spelling is "sympathetically."

47. A
Explanation: The subject of this sentence, "a team," is singular, so the verb also should be singular.

48. B
Explanation: This sentence is in the past tense so the phrasal verb should also be in the past tense.

49. A
Explanation: The correct spelling is "believes."

50. B
Explanation: The correct spelling is "presents."

51. D
Explanation: The correct spelling is "authority."

52. A

Explanation: The correct spelling is "traveled."

53. C

Explanation: The word "precipitous" means "steep."

54. B

Explanation: The word "obscure" means "unclear" and "difficult to understand."

55. C

Explanation: The word "remiss" means "negligent or forgetful."

Practice Test #2

Reading

DIRECTIONS: The reading practice test you are about to take is multiple-choice with only one correct answer per question. Read each test item and circle your answer on the answer sheet below. When you have completed the practice test, you may check your answers with the answers on the answer key following the test.

Answer Sheet

1.	a	b	c	d		21.	a	b	c	d
2.	a	b	c	d		22.	a	b	c	d
3.	a	b	c	d		23.	a	b	c	d
4.	a	b	c	d		24.	a	b	c	d
5.	a	b	c	d		25.	a	b	c	d
6.	a	b	c	d		26.	a	b	c	d
7.	a	b	c	d		27.	a	b	c	d
8.	a	b	c	d		28.	a	b	c	d
9.	a	b	c	d		29.	a	b	c	d
10.	a	b	c	d		30.	a	b	c	d
11.	a	b	c	d		31.	a	b	c	d
12.	a	b	c	d		32.	a	b	c	d
13.	a	b	c	d		33.	a	b	c	d
14.	a	b	c	d		34.	a	b	c	d
15.	a	b	c	d		35.	a	b	c	d
16.	a	b	c	d		36.	a	b	c	d
17.	a	b	c	d		37.	a	b	c	d
18.	a	b	c	d		38.	a	b	c	d
19.	a	b	c	d		39.	a	b	c	d
20.	a	b	c	d		40.	a	b	c	d

Reading Test

Read the passage below and answer questions 1-4.

It could be argued that all American war movies take as their governing paradigm that of the Western, and that we, as viewers, don't think critically enough about this fact. The virtuous hero in the white hat, the evil villain in the black hat, the community threatened by violence; these are the obvious elements of the paradigm. In addition, the hero is highly skilled at warfare, though reluctant to use it, the community is made up of morally upstanding citizens, and there is no place for violence in the community: the hero himself must leave the community he has saved once the battle is complete. This way of seeing the world has soaked into our storytelling of battle and conflict. It's hard to find a U.S.-made war movie that, for example, presents the enemy as complex and potentially fighting a legitimate cause, or that presents the hero (usually the U.S.) as anything other than supremely morally worthy. It is important to step back and think about the assumptions and frameworks that shape the stories we're exposed to; if we're careless and unquestioning, we absorb biases and world views with which we may not agree.

1. The primary purpose of this passage is to:
    a. analyze an interesting feature of American cinema.
    b. refute the Western paradigm.
    c. suggest a way that war movies could be made better.
    d. suggest that viewers think critically about underlying assumptions in the movies we watch.

2. The author claims that it is hard to find a U.S. made movie that "presents the hero (usually the U.S.) as anything other than supremely morally worthy." Does the author imply that she:
    a. believes the hero should always appear to be morally worthy.
    b. believes the hero should never appear to be morally worthy.
    c. believes the hero should be more nuanced and less unconditionally good.
    d. believes the hero is an uninteresting character.

3. Which of the following is <u>not</u> an example given by the author of an element of the Western paradigm:
    a. Hero highly skilled at warfare
    b. Evil villain in black hat
    c. Everyone riding horses
    d. Community made up of upstanding citizens

4. Which of the following is part of the world view, with which we may not agree, that the author implies we might absorb from these movies if we're careless and unquestioning:
    a. Enemies of the U.S. do not ever fight for legitimate causes.
    b. The community is morally bankrupt.
    c. The U.S. is complex.
    d. The U.S. is not skilled at warfare.

Read the passage below to answer questions 5-8.

It is most likely that you have never had diphtheria. You probably don't even know anyone who has suffered from this disease. In fact, you may not even know what diphtheria is. Similarly, diseases like whooping cough, measles, mumps, and rubella may all be unfamiliar to you. In the nineteenth and early twentieth centuries, these illnesses struck hundreds of thousands of people in the United States each year, mostly children, and tens of thousands of people died. The names of these diseases were frightening household words. Today, they are all but forgotten. That change happened largely because of vaccines.

You probably have been vaccinated against diphtheria. You may even have been exposed to the bacterium that causes it, but the vaccine prepared your body to fight off the disease so quickly that you were unaware of the infection. Vaccines take advantage of your body's natural ability to learn how to combat many disease-causing germs, or microbes. What's more, your body remembers how to protect itself from the microbes it has encountered before. Collectively, the parts of your body that remember and repel microbes are called the immune system. Without the proper functioning of the immune system, the simplest illness—even the common cold—could quickly turn deadly.

On average, your immune system needs more than a week to learn how to fight off an unfamiliar microbe. Sometimes, that isn't enough time. Strong microbes can spread through your body faster than the immune system can fend them off. Your body often gains the upper hand after a few weeks, but in the meantime you are sick. Certain microbes are so virulent that they can overwhelm or escape your natural defenses. In those situations, vaccines can make all the difference.

Traditional vaccines contain either parts of microbes or whole microbes that have been altered so that they don't cause disease. When your immune system confronts these harmless versions of the germs, it quickly clears them from your body. In other words, vaccines trick your immune system in order to teach your body important lessons about how to defeat its opponents.

5. What is the main idea of the passage?
    a. The nineteenth and early twentieth centuries were a dark period for medicine.
    b. You have probably never had diphtheria.
    c. Traditional vaccines contain altered microbes.
    d. Vaccines help the immune system function properly.

6. Which statement is *not* a detail from the passage?
    a. Vaccines contain microbe parts or altered microbes.
    b. The immune system typically needs a week to learn how to fight a new disease.
    c. The symptoms of disease do not emerge until the body has learned how to fight the microbe.
    d. A hundred years ago, children were at the greatest risk of dying from now-treatable diseases.

7. What is the meaning of the word *virulent* as it is used in the third paragraph?
    a. tiny
    b. malicious
    c. contagious
    d. annoying

8. What is the author's primary purpose in writing the essay?
    a. to entertain
    b. to persuade
    c. to inform
    d. to analyze

Read the passage below to answer questions 9-12.

The federal government regulates dietary supplements through the United States Food and Drug Administration (FDA). The regulations for dietary supplements are not the same as those for prescription or over-the-counter drugs. In general, the regulations for dietary supplements are less strict.

To begin with, a manufacturer does not have to prove the safety and effectiveness of a dietary supplement before it is marketed. A manufacturer is permitted to say that a dietary supplement addresses a nutrient deficiency, supports health, or is linked to a particular body function (such as immunity), if there is research to support the claim. Such a claim must be followed by the words "This statement has not been evaluated by the Food and Drug Administration. This product is not intended to diagnose, treat, cure, or prevent any disease."

Also, manufacturers are expected to follow certain good manufacturing practices (GMPs) to ensure that dietary supplements are processed consistently and meet quality standards. Requirements for GMPs went into effect in 2008 for large manufacturers and are being phased in for small manufacturers through 2010.

Once a dietary supplement is on the market, the FDA monitors safety and product information, such as label claims and package inserts. If it finds a product to be unsafe, it can take action against the manufacturer and/or distributor and may issue a warning or require that the product be removed from the marketplace. The Federal Trade Commission (FTC) is responsible for regulating product advertising; it requires that all information be truthful and not misleading.

The federal government has taken legal action against a number of dietary supplement promoters or Web sites that promote or sell dietary supplements because they have made false or deceptive statements about their products or because marketed products have proven to be unsafe.

9. What is the main idea of the passage?
    a. Manufacturers of dietary supplements have to follow good manufacturing practices.
    b. The FDA has a special program for regulating dietary supplements.
    c. The federal government prosecutes those who mislead the general public.
    d. The FDA is part of the federal government.

10. Which statement is *not* a detail from the passage?
    a. Promoters of dietary supplements can make any claims that are supported by research.
    b. GMP requirements for large manufacturers went into effect in 2008.
    c. Product advertising is regulated by the FTc.
    d. The FDA does not monitor products after they enter the market.

11. What is the meaning of the phrase *phased in* as it is used in the third paragraph?
    a. stunned into silence
    b. confused
    c. implemented in stages
    d. legalized

12. What is the meaning of the word *deceptive* as it is used in the fifth paragraph?
    a. misleading
    b. malicious
    c. illegal
    d. irritating

Questions 13- 17 refer to the following passage:

Tips for Eating Calcium Rich Foods
- Include milk as a beverage at meals. Choose fat-free or low-fat milk.
- If you usually drink whole milk, switch gradually to fat-free milk to lower saturated fat and calories. Try reduced fat (2%), then low-fat (1%), and finally fat-free (skim).
- If you drink cappuccinos or lattes—ask for them with fat-free (skim) milk.
- Add fat-free or low-fat milk instead of water to oatmeal and hot cereals
- Use fat-free or low-fat milk when making condensed cream soups (such as cream of tomato).
- Have fat-free or low-fat yogurt as a snack.
- Make a dip for fruits or vegetables from yogurt.
- Make fruit-yogurt smoothies in the blender.
- For dessert, make chocolate or butterscotch pudding with fat-free or low-fat milk.
- Top cut-up fruit with flavored yogurt for a quick dessert.
- Top casseroles, soups, stews, or vegetables with shredded low-fat cheese.
- Top a baked potato with fat-free or low-fat yogurt.

For those who choose not to consume milk products
- If you avoid milk because of lactose intolerance, the most reliable way to get the health benefits of milk is to choose lactose-free alternatives within the milk group, such as cheese, yogurt, or lactose-free milk, or to consume the enzyme lactase before consuming milk products.
- Calcium choices for those who do not consume milk products include:
    o Calcium fortified juices, cereals, breads, soy beverages, or rice beverages
    o Canned fish (sardines, salmon with bones) soybeans and other soy products, some other dried beans, and some leafy greens.

13. According to the passage, how can you lower saturated fat and calories in your diet?
    a. Add fat-free milk to oatmeal instead of water.
    b. Switch to fat-free milk.
    c. Drink calcium-fortified juice.
    d. Make yogurt dip.

14. What device does the author use to organize the passage?
    a. headings
    b. captions
    c. diagrams
    d. labels

15. How much fat does reduced fat milk contain?
    a. 0 percent
    b. 1 percent
    c. 2 percent
    d. 3 percent

16. Which of the following is true about calcium rich foods?
    I.   Canned salmon with bones contains calcium.
    II.   Cheese is a lactose-free food.
    III. Condensed soup made with water is a calcium rich food.
    a. I only
    b. I and II only
    c. II and III only
    d. III only

17. What information should the author include to help clarify information in the passage?
    a. The fat content of yogurt.
    b. How much calcium is in fortified juice.
    c. Which leafy greens contain calcium.
    d. The definition of lactose intolerance.

For each of the words below, pick the answer choice that most closely means the same thing.

18. exacerbate
    a. implicate
    b. aggravate
    c. heal
    d. decondition

19. repugnant
    a. destructive
    b. selective
    c. collective
    d. offensive

20. offsetting
    a. compensatory
    b. defensive
    c. untoward
    d. confused

21. flaccid
    a. defended
    b. limp
    c. slender
    d. outdated

22. belligerent
    a. retired
    b. sardonic
    c. pugnacious
    d. acclimated

23. insidious
    a. stealthy
    b. deadly
    c. collapsed
    d. new

Use the passage below to answer questions 24-28.

Daylight Saving Time (DST) is the practice of changing clocks so that afternoons have more daylight and mornings have less. Clocks are adjusted forward one hour in the spring and one hour backward in the fall. The main purpose of the change is to make better use of daylight.

DST began with the goal of conservation. Benjamin Franklin suggested it as a method of saving on candles. It was used during both World Wars to save energy for military needs. Although DST's potential to save energy was a primary reason behind its implementation, research into its effects on energy conservation are contradictory and unclear.

Beneficiaries of DST include all activities that can benefit from more sunlight after working hours, such as shopping and sports. A 1984 issue of *Fortune* magazine estimated that a seven-week extension of DST would yield an additional $30 million for 7-Eleven stores. Public safety may be increased by the use of DST: some research suggests that traffic fatalities may be reduced when there is additional afternoon sunlight.

On the other hand, DST complicates timekeeping and some computer systems. Tools with built-in time-keeping functions such as medical devices can be affected negatively. Agricultural and evening entertainment interests have historically opposed DST.

DST can affect health, both positively and negatively. It provides more afternoon sunlight in which to get exercise. It also impacts sunlight exposure; this is good for getting vitamin D, but bad in that it can increase skin cancer risk. DST may also disrupt sleep.

Today, daylight saving time has been adopted by more than one billion people in about 70 countries. DST is generally not observed in countries near the equator because sunrise times do not vary much there. Asia and Africa do not generally observe it. Some countries, such as Brazil, observe it only in some regions.

DST can lead to peculiar situations. One of these occurred in November, 2007 when a woman in North Carolina gave birth to one twin at 1:32 a.m. and, 34 minutes later, to the second twin. Because of DST and the time change at 2:00 a.m., the second twin was officially born at 1:06, 26 minutes earlier than her brother.

24. According to the passage, what is the main purpose of DST?
    a. To increase public safety
    b. To benefit retail businesses
    c. To make better use of daylight
    d. To promote good health

25. Which of the following is not mentioned in the passage as a negative effect of DST?
   a. Energy conservation
   b. Complications with time keeping
   c. Complications with computer systems
   d. Increased skin cancer risk

26. The article states that DST involves:
   a. Adjusting clocks forward one hour in the spring and the fall.
   b. Adjusting clocks backward one hour in the spring and the fall.
   c. Adjusting clocks forward in the fall and backward in the spring.
   d. Adjusting clocks forward in the spring and backward in the fall.

27. In what region does the article state DST is observed only in some regions?
   a. The equator
   b. Asia
   c. Africa
   d. Brazil

28. According to the passage, a 1984 magazine article estimated that a seven-week extension of DST would provide 7-Eleven stores with an extra $30 million. Approximately how much extra money is that per week of the extension?
   a. 42,000
   b. 420,000
   c. 4,200,000
   d. 42,000,000

Questions 29-32 are based on the following (2) passages.

Passage 1:

Fairy tales, fictional stories that involve magical occurrences and imaginary creatures like trolls, elves, giants, and talking animals, are found in similar forms throughout the world. This occurs when a story with an origin in a particular location spreads geographically to, over time, far-flung lands. All variations of the same story must logically come from a single source. As language, ideas, and goods travel from place to place through the movement of peoples, stories that catch human imagination travel as well through human retelling.

Passage 2:

Fairy tales capture basic, fundamental human desires and fears. They represent the most essential form of fictionalized human experience: the bad characters are pure evil, the good characters are pure good, the romance of royalty (and of commoners becoming royalty) is celebrated, etc. Given the nature of the fairy tale genre, it is not surprising that many different cultures come up with similar versions of the same essential story.

29. On what point would the authors of both passages agree?
    a. Fairy tales share a common origin.
    b. The same fairy tale may develop independently in a number of different cultures.
    c. There are often common elements in fairy tales from different cultures.
    d. Fairy tales capture basic human fears.

30. What does the "nature of the fairy tale genre" refer to in Passage 2?
    a. The representation of basic human experience
    b. Good characters being pure good and bad characters being pure evil
    c. Different cultures coming up with similar versions of the same story
    d. Commoners becoming royalty

31. Which of the following is not an example of something the author of Passage 1 claims travels from place to place through human movement?
    a. Fairy tales
    b. Language
    c. Ideas
    d. Foods

32. Which of the following is not an example of something that the author of Passage 1 states might be found in a fairy tale?
    a. Trolls
    b. Witches
    c. Talking animals
    d. Giants

Questions 33-34 *refer to the following passage*

What outdoorsy, family adventure can you have on a hot, summer day? How about spelunking? If you live in an area that is anywhere near a guided, lit cave, find out the hours of operation and hit the road towards it as soon as you can. Hitch up the double jogging stroller and make your way out into the wilderness, preferably with a guide, and discover the wonders of the cool, dark earth even while it is sweltering hot in the outside world. It will be 58 degrees in that cave, and you can explore inside for as long as you please. Best part? The absolutely awesome naps that the kids will take after such an exciting adventure! Be sure to bring:
- Bottled water
- Light-up tennis shoes if you have them (they look fabulous in the dark)
- Flashlights or glow sticks just for fun
- Jackets
- Changes of clothes in case of getting muddy and/or dirty

33. Based on the information given, what is spelunking?
    a. going in a cave
    b. an outdoor adventure
    c. walking with a double stroller
    d. a hot, summer day

34. Given the style of writing for the passage, which of the following magazines would be the best fit for this article?
    a. *Scientific Spelunking*
    b. *Family Fun Days*
    c. *Technical Caving in America*
    d. *Mud Magazine*

Questions 35-36 *refer to the following passage*

For lunch, she likes ham and cheese (torn into bites), yogurt, raisins, applesauce, peanut butter sandwiches in the fridge drawer, or any combo of these. She's not a huge eater. Help yourself too. Bread is on counter if you want to make a sandwich.

It's fine if you want to go somewhere, leave us a note of where you are. Make sure she's buckled and drive carefully! Certain fast food places are fun if they have playgrounds and are indoors. It's probably too hot for playground, but whatever you want to do is fine. Take a sippy cup of water and a diaper wherever you go. There's some money here for you in case you decide to go out for lunch with her.

As for nap, try after lunch. She may not sleep, but try anyway. Read her a couple of books first, put cream on her mosquito bites (it's in the den on the buffet), then maybe rock in her chair. Give her a bottle of milk, and refill as needed, but don't let her drink more than 2 ½ bottles of milk or she'll throw up. Turn on music in her room, leave her in crib with a dry diaper and bottle to try to sleep. She likes a stuffed animal too. Try for 30-45 minutes. You may have to start the tape again. If she won't sleep, that's fine. We just call it "rest time" on those days that naps won't happen.

35. To whom is this passage probably being written?
    a. a mother
    b. a father
    c. a babysitter
    d. a nurse

36. You can assume the writer of the passage is:
    a. a mom
    b. a dad
    c. a teacher
    d. a parent

Volleyball is easy to learn and fun to play in a physical education class. With just one net and one ball, an entire class can participate. The object of the game is to get the ball over the net and onto the ground on the other side. At the same time, all players should be in the ready position to keep the ball from hitting the ground on their own side. After the ball has been served, the opposing team may have three hits to get the ball over the net to the other side. Only the serving team may score. If the receiving team wins the volley, the referee calls, "side out" and the receiving team wins the serve. Players should rotate positions so that everyone gets a chance to serve. A game is played to 15 points, but the winning team must win by two points. That means if the score is 14 to 15, the play continues until one team wins by two. A volleyball match consists of three games. The winner of the match is the team that wins two of the three games.

37. Who can score in a volleyball game?
    a. the receiving team
    b. the serving team
    c. either team
    d. there is no score

38. How many people can participate in a volleyball game?
    a. 14
    b. 15
    c. half of a class
    d. an entire class

39. What is something that a referee might call in a volleyball game?
    a. "side out"
    b. "time out"
    c. "out of order"
    d. "be careful"

40. What equipment is needed for volleyball?
    a. a referee, a goal, a ball
    b. a goal, a ball, a net
    c. a net, a ball
    d. two balls, one net

Mathematics

DIRECTIONS: The mathematics practice test you are about to take is multiple-choice with only one correct answer per question. Read each test item and circle your answer on the answer sheet below. When you have completed the practice test, you may check your answers with the answers on the answer key following the test.

Answer Sheet

1.	a	b	c	d		24.	a	b	c	d
2.	a	b	c	d		25.	a	b	c	d
3.	a	b	c	d		26.	a	b	c	d
4.	a	b	c	d		27.	a	b	c	d
5.	a	b	c	d		28.	a	b	c	d
6.	a	b	c	d		29.	a	b	c	d
7.	a	b	c	d		30.	a	b	c	d
8.	a	b	c	d		31.	a	b	c	d
9.	a	b	c	d		32.	a	b	c	d
10.	a	b	c	d		33.	a	b	c	d
11.	a	b	c	d		34.	a	b	c	d
12.	a	b	c	d		35.	a	b	c	d
13.	a	b	c	d		36.	a	b	c	d
14.	a	b	c	d		37.	a	b	c	d
15.	a	b	c	d		38.	a	b	c	d
16.	a	b	c	d		39.	a	b	c	d
17.	a	b	c	d		40.	a	b	c	d
18.	a	b	c	d		41.	a	b	c	d
19.	a	b	c	d		42.	a	b	c	d
20.	a	b	c	d		43.	a	b	c	d
21.	a	b	c	d		44.	a	b	c	d
22.	a	b	c	d		45.	a	b	c	d
23.	a	b	c	d						

Mathematics Test

1. A man decided to buy new furniture from Futuristic Furniture for $2600. Futuristic Furniture gave the man two choices: pay the entire amount in one payment with cash, or pay $1000 as a down payment and $120 per month for two full years in the financial plan. If the man chooses the financial plan, how much more would he pay?
   a. $1480 more
   b. $1280 more
   c. $1600 more
   d. $2480 more

2. What is the value of r in the following equation?
   $29 + r = 420$
   a. $r = 29/420$
   b. $r = 420/29$
   c. $r = 391$
   d. $r = 449$

3. If 35% of a paycheck was deducted for taxes and 4% for insurance, what is the total percent taken out of the paycheck?
   a. 20%
   b. 31%
   c. 39%
   d. 42%

4. In the year 2000, 35% of the company sales were in electronics. The table below shows how electronic sales have changed for the company over the years. Find the percent of electronics sold in 2005.

Years	Change
2000 - 2001	-2
2001 - 2002	-1
2002 - 2003	+6
2003 - 2004	-1
2004 - 2005	+2

   a. 2%
   b. 11%
   c. 39%
   d. 42%

5. A woman wants to stack two small bookcases beneath a window that is 26½ inches from the floor. The larger bookcase is 14½ inches tall. The other bookcase is 8¾ inches tall. How tall with the two bookcases be when they are stacked together?
   a. 12 inches tall
   b. 23¼ inches tall
   c. 35¼ inches tall
   d. 41 inches tall

6. Solve for *y* in the following equation if *x* = -3

y = *x* + 5

 a. *y* = -2
 b. *y* = 2
 c. *y* = 3
 d. *y* = 8

7. Put the following integers in order from greatest to least:

-52, 16, -12, 14, 8, -5, 0

 a. -52, 16, -12, 14, 8, -5, 0
 b. 0, -5, 8, -12, 14, 16, -52
 c. -5, -12, -52, 0, 8, 14, 16
 d. 16, 14, 8, 0, -5, -12, -52

8. If number *x* is subtracted from 27, the result is -5. What is number *x*?

 a. 22
 b. 25
 c. 32
 d. 35

9. What is the simplest way to write the following expression?

 5x – 2y + 4x + y

 a. $9x - y$
 b. $9x - 3y$
 c. $9x + 3y$
 d. $x ; y$

10. Find the sum.

$(3x^2 + x + 3) + 8x^2 + 5x + 16$

 a. $7x^2 + 29 x^2$
 b. $11x^2 + 6x + 19$
 c. 30x + 19
 d. $(3x^2 + 3x) + 13x^2 + 16$

11. What is the perimeter of the following figure?

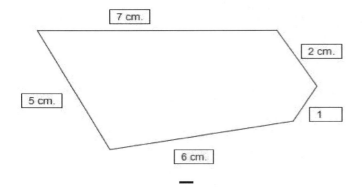

7 cm.

2 cm.

5 cm.

1

6 cm.

a. 15cm
b. 18cm
c. 21 cm
d. 36cm

12. To begin making her soup, Jennifer added four containers of chicken broth with 1 liter of water into the pot. Each container of chicken broth contains 410 milliliters. How much liquid is in the pot?
a. 1.64 liters
b. 2.64 liters
c. 5.44 liters
d. 6.12 liters

13. According to the table below, which snack is made with no more than 4 grams of sugar and between 4-6 grams of carbohydrates?

Snack (amount per serving)	Grams of Sugar per Serving	Grams of Carbohydrates per Serving
Snappy Cookies (3)	6	8
Snappy Crackers (8)	6	4
Snappy Cheese (2)	0	0
Snappy Twisters (4)	4	5
Snappy Chews (20)	0	8

a. Snappy Cookies
b. Snappy Crackers
c. Snappy Cheese
d. Snappy Twisters

14. Which of the following fractions is halfway between 2/5 and 4/9?
a. 2/3
b. 2/20
c. 17/40
d. 19/45

15. Which of the following is the largest number?
    a. 1/2
    b. 3/8
    c. 7/16
    d. 13/54

16. Of the following expressions, which is equal to $6\sqrt{10}$?
    a. 36
    b. $\sqrt{600}$
    c. $\sqrt{360}$
    d. $\sqrt{6}$

17. Which number equals 2^{-3}?
    a. ½
    b. ¼
    c. 1/8
    d. 1/16

18. What is the average of $\dfrac{7}{5}$ and 1.4 ?

    a. 5.4
    b. 1.4
    c. 2.4
    d. 7.4

19. Two numbers are said to be reciprocal if their product equals 1. Which of the following represents the reciprocal of the variable x?
    a. $x - 1$
    b. $\dfrac{1}{x}$
    c. x^{-1}
    d. Both B and c.

20. A taxi service charges $5.50 for the first 1/5th of a mile, $1.50 for each additional 1/5th of a mile, and 20¢ per minute of waiting time. Joan took a cab from her place to a flower shop 8 miles away, where she bought a bouquet, then another 3.6 miles to her mother's place. The driver had to wait 9 minutes while she bought the bouquet. What was the fare?
    a. $20
    b. $120.20
    c. $92.80
    d. $91

21. Which of the following expressions is equivalent to the equation $3x^2 + 4x - 15$?
    a. $(x - 3)(x + 5)$
    b. $(x + 5)(3 + x^2)$
    c. $x(3x + 4 - 15)$
    d. $(x + 3)(3x - 5)$

- 73 -

22. Prizes are to be awarded to the best pupils in each class of an elementary school. The number of students in each grade is shown in the table, and the school principal wants the number of prizes awarded in each grade to be proportional to the number of students. If there are twenty prizes, how many should go to fifth grade students?

Grade	1	2	3	4	5
Students	35	38	38	33	36

    a. 5
    b. 4
    c. 7
    d. 3

23. Which of the following numbers is a prime number?
    a. 15
    b. 11
    c. 33
    d. 4

24. Which of the following expressions is equivalent to $3(\frac{6x-3}{3})-3(9x+9)$?
    a. $-3(7x+10)$
    b. -3x +6
    c. $(x+3)(x-3)$
    d. $3x^2-9$

25. Evaluate the expression $(x-2y)^2$ where x = 3 and y = 2.
    a. -1
    b. +1
    c. +4
    d. -2

26. Bob decides to go into business selling lemonade. He buys a wooden stand for $45 and sets it up outside his house. He figures that the cost of lemons, sugar, and paper cups for each glass of lemonade sold will be 10¢. Which of these expressions describes his cost for making g glasses of lemonade?
    a. $\$45 + \$0.1 \times g$
    b. $\$44.90 \times g$
    c. $\$44.90 \times g + 10$¢
    d. $90

27. Which of the following expressions is equivalent to $(3x^{-2})^3$?
    a. $9x^{-6}$
    b. $9x^{-8}$
    c. $27x^{-8}$
    d. $27x^{-4}$

28. Sally wants to buy a used truck for her delivery business. Truck A is priced at $450 and gets 25 miles per gallon. Truck B costs $650 and gets 35 miles per gallon. If gasoline costs $4 per gallon, how many miles must Sally drive to make truck B the better buy?
   a. 500
   b. 7500
   c. 1750
   d. 4375

29. Given the equation $\dfrac{3}{y-5} = \dfrac{15}{y+4}$, what is the value of y?
   a. 45
   b. 54
   c. $\dfrac{29}{4}$
   d. $\dfrac{4}{29}$

30. Which of the following expressions is equivalent to $(a)(a)(a)(a)(a)$ for all values of a, positive or negative?
   a. $5a$
   b. a^{-5}
   c. $a^{-\frac{1}{5}}$
   d. a^{5}

31.

English-Metric Equivalents	
1 meter	1.094 yard
2.54 centimeter	1 inch
1 kilogram	2.205 pound
1 liter	1.06 quart

A sailboat is 19 meters long. What is its length in inches?
   a. 254
   b. 1094
   c. 4826
   d. 748

Questions 32 and 33 are based upon the following table:

Kyle bats third in the batting order for the Badgers baseball team. The table shows the number of hits that Kyle had in each of 7 consecutive games played during one week in July.

Day of Week	Number of Hits
Monday	1
Tuesday	2
Wednesday	3
Thursday	1
Friday	1
Saturday	4
Sunday	2

32. What is the mode of the numbers in the distribution shown in the table?
   a. 1
   b. 2
   c. 3
   d. 4

33. What is the mean of the numbers in the distribution shown in the table?
   a. 1
   b. 2
   c. 3
   d. 4

34. $(2a^2b - 3c^3)(3a^3b + 4c) =$
   a. $5a^6b^2 + 12c^4 - 9a^3bc^3 - 12c^4$
   b. $5a^5b^2 + 8a^2bc - 9a^3bc^3 + 12c^4$
   c. $6a^5b^2 + 8a^2bc - 9a^3bc^3 + 12c^4$
   d. $6a^5b^2 + 8a^2bc - 9a^3bc^3 - 12c^4$

Questions 35-40 refer to the following chart:

Profile of Staff at Mercy Hospital in City X and Mercy Hospital in City Y
Total Combined Staff: 433

City X (250)	Profession	City Y (183)
74	Doctor	55
121	Registered Nurse	87
14	Administrator	9
15	Maintenance	11
6	Pharmacist	5
4	Radiologist	2
2	Physical Therapist	2
1	Speech Pathologist	1
13	Other	11
	Gender	
153	Male	93
97	Female	90
	Age	
24	Youngest	22
73	Oldest	77
	Ethnicity	
51	African American	42
50	Asian American	27
45	Hispanic American	35
47	Caucasian	37
57	Other	42
	Years on Staff	
64	0-5 32	
63	5-10	41
57	10-15	67
47	15-20	30
14	20-25	19
5	More than 25	5
	Number of Patient Complaints	
202	0	161
43	1-4	21
5	5-10	1
0	More than 10	0

35. Approximately what percentage of City X hospital staff are doctors?
    a. 15
    b. 20
    c. 25
    d. 30

36. If a speech pathologist in City Y has 6 patient complaints, how many doctors there have five or more patient complaints?
   a. 0
   b. 1
   c. 21
   d. 55

37. Which percentage is greatest?
   a. The percentage of Asian Americans to staff as a whole in City X?
   b. The percentage of staff members who have been on staff 10-15 years to staff as a whole in City X?
   c. The percentage of Doctors to staff as a whole in City X and City Y?
   d. The percentage of staff with 1-4 complaints to staff as a whole in City Y?

38. If all Caucasian staff members in City Y have been on staff between 5-10 years, how many non-Caucasian staff members in City Y have been on staff 5-10 years?
   a. 0
   b. 4
   c. 37
   d. 41

39. Approximately what percentage more staff members in City Y are female than in City X?
   a. 5
   b. 10
   c. 15
   d. 20

40. According to the chart, the percentage of staff who have received zero complaints is
   a. greater in City X than in City Y
   b. greater in City Y than in City X
   c. the same in City X and in City Y
   d. growing in both City X and City Y

41. In the following inequality, solve for x.
$-4x + 8 \geq 48$
   a. $x \geq 10$
   b. $x \geq -10$
   c. $x \leq 10$
   d. $x \leq -10$

42. Two even integers and one odd integer are multiplied together. Which of the following could be their product?
   a. 3.75
   b. 9
   c. 16.2
   d. 24

43. There are 80 mg / 0.8 ml in Acetaminophen Concentrated Infant Drops. If the proper dosage for a four year old child is 240 mg, how many milliliters should the child receive?
    a. 0.8 ml
    b. 1.6 ml
    c. 2.4 ml
    d. 3.2 ml

44. Using the chart below, which equation describes the relationship between *x* and *y*?

    a. x = 3y
    b. y = 3x
    c. y = 1/3x
    d. x/y = 3

x	y
2	6
3	9
4	12
5	15

45. On a highway map, the scale indicates that 1 inch represents 45 miles. If the distance on the map is 3.2 inches, how far is the actual distance?
    a. 45 miles
    b. 54 miles
    c. 112 miles
    d. 144 miles

Science and Technical Reasoning

DIRECTIONS: The science and technical reasoning practice test you are about to take is multiple-choice with only one correct answer per question. Read each test item and circle your answer on the answer sheet below. When you have completed the practice test, you may check your answers with those on the answer key that follows the test.

Answer Sheet

1.	a	b	c	d
2.	a	b	c	d
3.	a	b	c	d
4.	a	b	c	d
5.	a	b	c	d
6.	a	b	c	d
7.	a	b	c	d
8.	a	b	c	d
9.	a	b	c	d
10.	a	b	c	d
11.	a	b	c	d
12.	a	b	c	d
13.	a	b	c	d
14.	a	b	c	d
15.	a	b	c	d
16.	a	b	c	d
17.	a	b	c	d
18.	a	b	c	d
19.	a	b	c	d
20.	a	b	c	d
21.	a	b	c	d
22.	a	b	c	d
23.	a	b	c	d
24.	a	b	c	d
25.	a	b	c	d
26.	a	b	c	d
27.	a	b	c	d
28.	a	b	c	d
29.	a	b	c	d
30.	a	b	c	d

Science and Technical Reasoning Test

1. A normal human sperm must contain:
   a. An X chromosome
   b. A Y chromosome
   c. 23 chromosomes
   d. B and C

2. During the process of oogenesis, primary oocytes produce:
   a. Sperm
   b. Eggs
   c. Oogonia
   d. Stem cells

3. In an oxidation reaction:
   a. An oxidizing agent gains electrons.
   b. An oxidizing agent loses electrons.
   c. A reducing agent gains electrons.
   d. reducing agent loses electrons.

4. The digestion of starch begins:
   a. In the mouth
   b. In the stomach
   c. In the pylorus
   d. In the duodenum

5. A neuron consists of three main parts. These are:
   a. Effector, cell body, axon
   b. Dendrites, axon, cell body
   c. Dendrites, axon, receptor
   d. Synapse, axon, cell body

6. Of the following, the blood vessel containing the least-oxygenated blood is:
   a. The aorta
   b. The vena cava
   c. The pulmonary artery
   d. The capillaries

7. A Tsunami may be caused by:
   a. Earthquakes
   b. Volcanoes
   c. Landslides
   d. A, B, and C

8. All living organisms on Earth utilize:
   a. Oxygen
   b. Light
   c. Sexual reproduction
   d. A triplet genetic code

9. A cannon sits on top of a cliff 20 meters above an expanse of level ground. It fires a 5 kg
   cannonball horizontally (cannonball A) at 5 meters/second. At the same time, a second
   cannonball (cannonball B) is dropped from the same height. If air resistance is negligible, which
   cannonball will hit the ground first?
   Note: The gravitational acceleration due to the Earth is 9.8 m/sec².
   a. Cannonball A
   b. Cannonball B
   c. Both will hit the ground at the same time.
   d. It will depend upon the temperature.

10. If an organism is *AaBb*, which of the following combinations in the gametes is impossible?
    a. AB
    b. aa
    c. aB
    d. Ab

11. How does water affect the temperature of a living thing?
    a. Water increases temperature.
    b. Water keeps temperature stable.
    c. Water decreases temperature.
    d. Water does not affect temperature.

12. Which of the following is *not* a product of the Krebs cycle?
    a. carbon dioxide
    b. oxygen
    c. adenosine triphosphate (ATP)
    d. energy carriers

13. What kind of bond connects sugar and phosphate in DNA?
    a. hydrogen
    b. ionic
    c. covalent
    d. overt

14. What is the second part of an organism's scientific name?
    a. species
    b. phylum
    c. population
    d. kingdom

15. What is the name for a cell that does *not* contain a nucleus?
    a. eukaryote
    b. bacteria
    c. prokaryote
    d. cancer

16. Which of the following forms of water is the densest?
    a. liquid
    b. steam
    c. ice
    d. All forms of water have the same density.

17. What is the oxidation number of hydrogen in CaH_2?
    a. +1
    b. −1
    c. 0
    d. +2

18. Which of the following could be an empirical formula?
    a. C4H8
    b. C2H6
    c. CH
    d. C3H6

19. What is the name for the reactant that is entirely consumed by the reaction?
    a. limiting reactant
    b. reducing agent
    c. reaction intermediate
    d. reagent

20. What is the name for the horizontal rows of the periodic table?
    a. groups
    b. periods
    c. families
    d. sets

21. What is the mass (in grams) of 7.35 mol water?
    a. 10.7 g
    b. 18 g
    c. 132 g
    d. 180.6 g

22. What is 119°K in degrees Celsius?
    a. 32°C
    b. −154°C
    c. 154°C
    d. −32°C

23. How many different types of tissue are there in the human body?
   a. four
   b. six
   c. eight
   d. ten

24. What is the name of the outermost layer of skin?
   a. dermis
   b. epidermis
   c. subcutaneous tissue
   d. hypodermis

25. Which of the following structures has the lowest blood pressure?
   a. arteries
   b. arteriole
   c. venule
   d. vein

26. Which of the heart chambers is the most muscular?
   a. left atrium
   b. right atrium
   c. left ventricle
   d. right ventricle

27. Which part of the brain interprets sensory information?
   a. cerebrum
   b. hindbrain
   C cerebellum
   d. medulla oblongata

28. Which of the following proteins is produced by cartilage?
   a. actin
   b. estrogen
   c. collagen
   d. myosin

29. Which component of the nervous system is responsible for lowering the heart rate?
   a. central nervous system
   b. sympathetic nervous system
   c. parasympathetic nervous system
   d. distal nervous system

30. How much air does an adult inhale in an average breath?
   a. 500 mL
   b. 750 mL
   c. 1000 mL
   d. 1250 mL

English and Language Usage

DIRECTIONS: The English and language usage practice test you are about to take is multiple-choice with only one correct answer per question. Read each test item and circle your answer on the answer sheet below. When you have completed the practice test, you may check your answers with those answers on the answer key that follows the test.

Answer Sheet

1.	a	b	c	d		29.	a	b	c	d
2.	a	b	c	d		30.	a	b	c	d
3.	a	b	c	d		31.	a	b	c	d
4.	a	b	c	d		32.	a	b	c	d
5.	a	b	c	d		33.	a	b	c	d
6.	a	b	c	d		34.	a	b	c	d
7.	a	b	c	d		35.	a	b	c	d
8.	a	b	c	d		36.	a	b	c	d
9.	a	b	c	d		37.	a	b	c	d
10.	a	b	c	d		38.	a	b	c	d
11.	a	b	c	d		39.	a	b	c	d
12.	a	b	c	d		40.	a	b	c	d
13.	a	b	c	d		41.	a	b	c	d
14.	a	b	c	d		42.	a	b	c	d
15.	a	b	c	d		43.	a	b	c	d
16.	a	b	c	d		44.	a	b	c	d
17.	a	b	c	d		45.	a	b	c	d
18.	a	b	c	d		46.	a	b	c	d
19.	a	b	c	d		47.	a	b	c	d
20.	a	b	c	d		48.	a	b	c	d
21.	a	b	c	d		49.	a	b	c	d
22.	a	b	c	d		50.	a	b	c	d
23.	a	b	c	d		51.	a	b	c	d
24.	a	b	c	d		52.	a	b	c	d
25.	a	b	c	d		53.	a	b	c	d
26.	a	b	c	d		54.	a	b	c	d
27.	a	b	c	d		55.	a	b	c	d
28.	a	b	c	d						

English and Language Usage Test

Questions 1-15 pertain to the following passage. Read the passage and correct the underlined words or phrases.

Passage I

In 2001, 34% of the population of the United States was overweight. Problems of excessive weight (1)<u>would seem to be</u> associated with the wealth and (2)<u>more than sufficient</u> food supply. (3)<u>Much attention in recent years has been paid</u> to physical fitness and (4)<u>changing their diets</u> to become healthier. It seems logical that, with so much emphasis on health and nutrition, (5)<u>that</u> the solution to our nation's obesity problem would be in (6)<u>sight</u>. However, in a study of a population with moderate food insecurity, it was found that (7)<u>52%</u> were overweight. *Food insecurity* exists when the availability of nutritionally adequate and safe foods or the ability to acquire acceptable foods in socially acceptable ways is limited or uncertain. Over half of (8)the <u>United State's</u> population with a threat of hunger is overweight. Why would obesity be more prevalent among this group of people who have *fewer* resources?

Dieting and surgery do not address the problems of the economic groups with the most severe weight and nutrition problems. Surgery is expensive, and people with limited resources are (9)<u>still</u> not likely to buy expensive health foods when there are cheaper alternatives that satisfy (10)<u>your</u> hunger. The dollar menu at a fast food restaurant is certainly less expensive than preparing a well-balanced meal, (11)<u>and easier too</u>. Another reason for obesity in lower income groups is given by (12)<u>a theory called</u> the paycheck cycle theory. Most paychecks are distributed on a monthly basis, so if a family gets a paycheck, (13)<u>the family</u> will use these resources until they run out. Often money can be depleted before the next distribution. When this happens, there is an involuntary restriction of food. The hypothesis suggests (14)<u>that a</u> cycle of food restriction at the end of the month followed by bingeing that would promote weight gain. The main reasons for obesity and overweight in low-income groups (15)<u>would be</u> periodic food restriction and a poor diet because of financial restrictions.

Questions: Passage I

1.
   a. NO CHANGE
   b. are
   c. seem to be
   d. are not

2.
   a. NO CHANGE
   b. more, then sufficient
   c. more, than sufficient
   d. more-than-sufficient

3.
   a. NO CHANGE
   b. In recent years, much attention has been paid
   c. Much attention, in recent years, has been paid
   d. In recent years much attention

4.
   a. NO CHANGE
   b. diet
   c. changing diet there
   d. changing your diet
5.
   a. NO CHANGE
   b. OMIT the word
   c. for
   d. when
6.
   a. NO CHANGE
   b. site
   c. cyte
   d. cite
7.
   a. NO CHANGE
   b. 52% of them
   c. 52% of the population
   d. 52% of it
8.
   a. NO CHANGE
   b. United States's
   c. United States
   d. United State
9.
   a. NO CHANGE
   b. OMIT word
   c. often
   d. frequently
10.
   a. NO CHANGE
   b. OMIT word
   c. ones
   d. the
11.
   a. NO CHANGE
   b. and easier to
   c. and easier two
   d. and easier, too
12.
   a. NO CHANGE
   b. OMIT expression
   c. something called
   d. a hypothesis called
13.
   a. NO CHANGE
   b. OMIT expression
   c. they
   d. someone

14.
    a. NO CHANGE
    b. that
    c. that there is
    d. doing a
15.
    a. NO CHANGE
    b. are
    c. seem to be
    d. come from

Questions 16-30 pertain to the following passage. Read the passage and correct the underlined words or phrases.

Passage II
Volta Hall is a (16)<u>womens</u> residence located at the western side of campus. It is composed of a (17)<u>porters</u> lodge, a small chapel, a dining hall, a library, a small laundry service, a hair salon, a small (18)<u>convenient</u> store, and three residential buildings designated for students.

Volta Hall has a total of three entry points that (19)<u>accesses</u> the entire structure. Two of these entries are located on the sides of the dining hall and are left unlocked and unprotected throughout the day. In the evening, usually (20)<u>some time</u> shortly after seven o'clock, these (21)<u>entryways</u> are locked by Volta Hall personnel. This leaves only the main entry, which is located at the front of the hall, (22)<u>as the only way</u> for individuals entering and exiting the hall. No record is kept of students or other persons entering and exiting the building. No identification is required to receive room keys from the porters. Security is so lax that students <u>(23)have been known to even receive</u> more than one room key from the porters and (24)<u>even</u> grab keys from behind the desk without giving notice.

The main entrance is guarded by two porters 24 hours (25)<u>out of each day</u>. The porters are most alert during the morning and early afternoon. During the evening (26)<u>hours</u> and early morning, the porters can be found sleeping. The main entry is usually closed during the late evening and reopened in the morning. Although these doors are closed, individuals have been known to open the latches from the outside, without forcing them, to gain entry.

There are usually additional security guards on the second level. During the day, two security guards are (27)<u>on watch or lack there of</u>. These guards are elderly men who have been known to respond to incidents very slowly, have poor eyesight, are unarmed, (28)<u>and physically out of shape</u>. Throughout the day and most of the evening, these guards can be found asleep at their post. Only one guard is on duty during the evening hours. These men can be found periodically walking around the perimeter of the building "checking" on students. These tactics have been (29)<u>proven to be</u> ineffective (30)<u>toward</u> criminal incidents occurring within the hall.

Questions: Passage II

16.
  a. NO CHANGE
  b. woman's
  c. women's
  d. womens's

17.
  a. NO CHANGE
  b. porter
  c. porter's
  d. porters's

18.
  a. NO CHANGE
  b. OMIT word
  c. convenience
  d. connivance

19.
  a. NO CHANGE
  b. come into
  c. come in to
  d. provide access to

20.
  a. NO CHANGE
  b. OMIT expression
  c. sometimes
  d. a little

21.
  a. NO CHANGE
  b. entry ways
  c. door ways
  d. windows

22.
  a. NO CHANGE
  b. OMIT phrase
  c. as the way
  d. as the best way

23.
  a. NO CHANGE
  b. receive
  c. have even been known to receive
  d. get

24.
  a. NO CHANGE
  b. OMIT word
  c. even to
  d. to

25.
  a. NO CHANGE
  b. a day
  c. at a time
  d. on their shifts

26.
  a. NO CHANGE
  b. OMIT word
  c. entrance
  d. hour's

27.
  a. NO CHANGE
  b. on watch or lack thereof
  c. supposedly on watch
  d. not enough

28.
  a. NO CHANGE
  b. and out of shape
  c. and are physically out of shape
  d. and are out of shape

29.
  a. NO CHANGE
  b. OMIT expression
  c. proved to be
  d. tried to be

30.
  a. NO CHANGE
  b. OMIT word
  c. when it comes to
  d. in curbing

Answer the following items.

31. _____ screaming took the shopkeeper by surprise.
  a. We
  b. They
  c. Them
  d. Our

32. Janet called her _____ run after a squirrel.
  a. dog, who had
  b. dog that had
  c. dog, that had
  d. dog who had

33. Which word is used incorrectly in the following sentence?
The video store is on the way, so we should stop by and rent one.
   a. video
   b. way
   c. by
   d. one

34. Which word is *not* used correctly in the context of the following sentence?
There is no real distinction among the two treatment protocols recommended online.
   a. real
   b. among
   c. protocols
   d. online

Read the following weather forecast and answer questions 35 – 39.

(1) Kids and people need to spend more time outside on a daily basis. <u>Last Child in the Woods: Saving Our Children from Nature-Deficit Disorder</u> is by Richard Louv and who says that in the last 30 years kids have become increasingly removed from nature to their detriment. **(2)** A 1991 study found that the radius children are allowed to roam outside their homes has shrunk to 1/9 of what it was 20 years before.

(3) Very bad for their physical fitness and mental health. **(4)** One in 5 American children is obese—compared with one in 20 in the late 1960s—and nearly 8 million kids suffer from mental illnesses, including depression and attention deficit disorder. **(5)** He says playing in nature helps reduce stress, increase concentration and promote problem-solving, this can help kids with attention deficit disorder and many other problems.   Nature play can increase a child's self confidence and independence.

(6) Parents are scared to let kids play in the woods. **(7)** Parents are increasingly afraid of child abduction. **(8)** This is a terrible thing but actually very rare and fear of them should be balanced against the effect of fear on our daily lives.

(9) Kids play too many video games, watch too much television and are in the car for long stretches of time. **(10)** It is important to have the experience of wet feet and dirty hands and not just read about a frog, for example but to hold it in your hands.

(11) Parents and emphasize organized sports over imaginative play. **(12)** It's great that kids play so much organized sports now, but activity and physical play used to be what kids did with their free time, not twice a week for soccer practice.

35. Which version of the following portion of sentence 2 provides the most clarity? *"...is by Richard Louv and who says that in the last 30 years kids have become increasingly removed..."*
   a. is by Richard Louv and who says that in the last 30 years kids have become increasingly removed
   b. is by Richard Louv, who says that in the last 30 years kids have become increasingly removed
   c. is by Richard Louv and he says that in the last 30 years kids have become increasingly removed
   d. is by Richard Louv he says that in the last 30 years kids have become increasingly removed

36. Which of the following is the most succinct and clear way to re-write sentences 6 and 7?
   a. Parents are scared to let kids play in the woods. Parents are increasingly afraid of child abduction.
   b. Parents are scared to let kids play in the woods and are increasingly afraid of child abduction.
   c. Parents are scared to let kids play in the woods because they are increasingly afraid of child abduction.
   d. Parents are scared to let kids play in the woods so they are increasingly afraid of child abduction.

37. Which of the following represents the best version of sentence 3?
   a. Very bad for their physical fitness and mental health.
   b. It is very bad for their physical fitness and mental health.
   c. This is very bad for their physical fitness and mental health.
   d. This "Nature-Deficit Disorder" is very bad for their physical fitness and mental health.

38. Sentence 8 is poorly written. What can we infer the initial "This" of the sentence refers to?
   a. Parents
   b. Kids
   c. Play
   d. Child abduction

39. The paragraph that includes sentences 9 and 10 does not contain a clear point. Which of the following best describes what the author is likely trying to communicate in this paragraph?
   a. Nature is important.
   b. It is a problem that kids are increasingly entertained by technology, rather than by the sensory experience of nature.
   c. It is a problem that kids are increasingly lethargic.
   d. It is a problem that kids are removed from nature.

Read the passage below to answer questions 40 – 43.

Most people think that the Giant Sequoia (*Sequoiadendron giganteum*) is the largest living organism. This conifer grows mostly in groves located in the Sierra Nevada Mountains in California. The biggest single Giant Sequoia is called the General Sherman tree. The General Sherman is 250 feet tall and has a diameter of 24.75 feet at the bottom. The trunk of this massive tree weighs nearly 1400 tons. That's about the weight of 10 trains or 15 fully grown blue whales.

But some people do not think that labeling the Giant Sequoia as the largest living organism is correct. That is because the majority of the material that makes up a tree is made up of dead cells rather than living matter. In addition, there are other types of plants that reproduce in such a way that they are connected with roots under the ground, such as a grove of aspen trees or a field of goldenrod flowers. Some people think that these large, connected groves should be considered the largest organism. In any case, a Giant Sequoia is indeed a massive and beautiful sight to behold indeed.

40. Based on the context of this passage, what is a conifer?
    a. an animal
    b. a tree
    c. a flower
    d. a cell

41. Is the Giant Sequoia the largest organism?
    a. yes
    b. no
    c. some people think it is
    d. most people think so

42. Why do some people think that a grove of aspen trees should be considered the largest organism?
    a. because the trees are taller
    b. because the trees have a wider diameter
    c. because the grove is connected underneath the ground
    d. because there are more of them in the United States

43. What is the diameter of the General Sherman tree at the top?
    a. 15 feet
    b. 20 feet
    c. 24.75 feet
    d. this question cannot be answered from the information given.

Fill in the blanks for questions 44 through 48.

44. The attendant looked ____ at everything related to the problem.
    a. close
    b. closet
    c. closely
    d. closedly

45. He decided to buy a large coal furnace because he felt it would be _____ than a woodstove.
   a. more efficient
   b. efficienter
   c. more efficienter
   d. efficiency

46. After waking up, Dean eyed the cheesecake _____.
   a. hungry
   b. hungriest
   c. hungrily
   d. more hungry

47. A child is not yet old enough to know what is healthy for _____.
   a. him or her
   b. them
   c. it
   d. she or he

48. _____ went to the movies after having dinner at Lenny's.
   a. Her and I
   b. Her and me
   c. She and I
   d. She and me

49. Which word is *not* spelled correctly in the context of the following sentence?
Dr. Vargas was surprised that the prescription had effected Ron's fatigue so dramatically.
   a. surprised
   b. prescription
   c. effected
   d. fatigue

50. Which word is *not* spelled correctly in the context of the following sentence?
The climate hear is inappropriate for snow sports such as skiing.
   a. climate
   b. hear
   c. inappropriate
   d. skiing

51. Which word is *not* used correctly in the context of the following sentence?
Before you walk any further, beware of the approaching traffic.
   a. before
   b. further
   c. beware
   d. approaching

52. Which word is *not* used correctly in the context of the following sentence?
There is no real distinction among the two treatment protocols recommended online.
    a. real
    b. among
    c. protocols
    d. online

Choose the meaning of the underlined words in the sentences below.

53. Her concern for him was **sincere.**
    a. intense
    b. genuine
    c. brief
    d. misunderstood

54. He is a very **courteous** young man.
    a. handsome
    b. polite
    c. inconsiderate
    d. odd

55. Spanish is a difficult language to **comprehend**.
    a. learn
    b. speak
    c. understand
    d. appreciate

Answer Key

	Reading	Mathematics	Science	English
1	D	B	C	C
2	C	C	B	D
3	C	C	A	B
4	A	C	A	B
5	D	B	B	B
6	C	B	C	A
7	B	D	D	A
8	C	C	D	B
9	B	A	C	B
10	D	B	B	B
11	C	C	B	D
12	A	B	B	B
13	B	D	C	C
14	A	D	A	C
15	C	A	C	C
16	B	C	A	C
17	D	C	B	C
18	B	B	C	C
19	D	D	A	D
20	A	C	B	B
21	B	D	C	A
22	C	B	B	B
23	A	B	A	C
24	C	A	B	D
25	A	B	D	B
26	D	A	C	B
27	D	C	A	C
28	C	D	C	D
29	C	C	C	B
30	A	D	A	D
31	D	D		D
32	B	A		A
33	A	B		D
34	B	D		B
35	C	D		B
36	D	A		C
37	B	C		D
38	D	B		D
39	A	B		B
40	C	B		B
41		D		D
42		D		C
43		C		D
44		B		C

	Reading	Mathematics	Science	English
45		D		A
46				C
47				A
48				C
49				C
50				B
51				B
52				B
53				B
54				B
55				C

Reading Answer Explanations

1. D
Explanation: The point of the passage is to suggest that viewers should think more critically about assumptions and frameworks (such as the Western paradigm) that underlie the stories in movies they watch.

2. C
Explanation: The author recommends that viewers think more critically about frameworks that underlie stories in movies; she argues that, if not, viewers may absorb biases with which they do not agree. An example the author gives of that bias is that it is hard to find a movie in which the hero is not supremely morally worthy. The author's identification of this as a bias implies that she thinks it is not the right choice. Her comment about the difficulty of finding a portrayal of an enemy that allows the enemy to be complex suggests that the author believes that more nuance and less absolutes would be an improvement in the U.S. storytelling of war.

3. C
Explanation: The author said nothing about horseback riding.

4. A
Explanation: The author suggests that these movies rarely show enemies of the U.S. to be complex or fighting for a legitimate cause.

5. D
Explanation: The main idea of this passage is that vaccines help the immune system function properly. Identifying main ideas is one of the key skills tested by the reading comprehension exam. One of the common traps that many test-takers fall into is assuming that the first sentence of the passage will express the main idea. Although this will be true for some passages, often the author will use the first sentence to attract interest or to make an introductory, but not central, point. On this question, if you assume that the first sentence contains the main idea, you will mistakenly choose answer b. Finding the main idea of a passage requires patience and thoroughness; you cannot expect to know the main idea until you have read the entire passage. In this case, a diligent reading will show you that answer choices A, B, and C express details from the passage, but only answer choice D is a comprehensive summary of the author's message.

6. C
Explanation: This passage does not state that the symptoms of disease will not emerge until the body has learned to fight the disease. The reading comprehension section of the exam will include several questions that require you to identify details from a passage. The typical structure of these questions is to ask you to identify the answer choice that contains a detail not included in the passage. This question structure makes your work a little more difficult, because it requires you to confirm that the other three details are in the passage. In this question, the details expressed in answer choices A, B, and D are all explicit in the passage. The passage never states, however, that the symptoms of disease do not emerge until the body has learned how to fight the disease-causing microbe. On the contrary, the passage

implies that a person may become quite sick and even die before the body learns to effectively fight the disease.

7. B
Explanation: In the third paragraph, the word *virulent* means "malicious." The reading comprehension section of the exam will include several questions that require you to define a word as it is used in the passage. Sometimes the word will be one of those used in the vocabulary section of the exam; other times, the word in question will be a slightly difficult word used regularly in academic and professional circles. In some cases, you may already know the basic definition of the word. Nevertheless, you should always go back and look at the way the word is used in the passage. The exam will often include answer choices that are legitimate definitions for the given word, but which do not express how the word is used in the passage. For instance, the word *virulent* could in some circumstances mean contagious or annoying. However, since the passage is not talking about transfer of the disease and is referring to a serious illness, malicious is the more appropriate answer.

8. C
Explanation: The author's primary purpose in writing this essay is to inform. The reading comprehension section of the exam will include a few questions that ask you to determine the purpose of the author. The answer choices are always the same: The author's purpose is to entertain, to persuade, to inform, or to analyze. When an author is *writing to entertain*, he or she is not including a great deal of factual information; instead, the focus is on vivid language and interesting stories. *Writing to persuade* means "trying to convince the reader of something." When a writer is just trying to provide the reader with information, without any particular bias, he or she is *writing to inform*. Finally, *writing to analyze* means to consider a subject already well known to the reader. For instance, if the above passage took an objective look at the pros and cons of various approaches to fighting disease, we would say that the passage was a piece of analysis. Because the purpose of this passage is to present new information to the reader in an objective manner, however, it is clear that the author's intention is to inform.

9. B
Explanation: The main idea of the passage is that the Food and Drug Administration (FDA) has a special program for regulating dietary supplements. This passage has a straightforward structure: The author introduces his subject in the first paragraph and uses the four succeeding paragraphs to elaborate. All of the other possible answers are true statements from the passage but cannot be considered the main idea. One way to approach questions about the main idea is to take sentences at random from the passage and see which answer choice they could potentially support. The main idea should be strengthened or supported by most of the details from the passage.

10. D
Explanation: The passage never states that the Food and Drug Administration (FDA) ignores products after they enter the market. In fact, the entire fourth paragraph describes the steps taken by the FDA to regulate products once they are available for purchase. In some cases, questions of this type will contain answer choices that are directly contradictory. Here, for instance, answer choices A and B cannot be true if answer choice D is true. If there are at least two answer choices that contradict another answer choice, it is a safe bet that the contradicted answer choice cannot be correct. If you are at all uncertain about your logic, however, you should refer to the passage.

11. C
Explanation: In the third paragraph, the phrase *phased in* means "implemented in stages."
Do not be tempted by the similarity of this phrase to the word *fazed*, which can mean
"confused or stunned." The author is referring to manufacturing standards that have
already been implemented for large manufacturers and are in the process of being
implemented for small manufacturers. It would make sense, then, for these standards to be
implemented in *phases*: that is, to be *phased in*.

12. A
Explanation: In the fifth paragraph, the word *deceptive* means "misleading." The root of the
word *deceptive* is the same as for the words *deceive* and *deception*. Take a look at the context
in which the word is used. The author states that the FDA prevents certain kinds of
advertising. It would be somewhat redundant for the author to mean that the FDA prevents
illegal advertising; this goes without saying. At the same time, it is unlikely that the FDA
spends its time trying to prevent merely *irritating* advertising; the persistent presence of
such advertising makes this answer choice inappropriate. Left with a choice between
malicious and *misleading* advertising, it makes better sense to choose the latter, since being
mean and nasty would be a bad technique for selling a product. It is common, however, for
an advertiser to deliberately mislead the consumer.

13. B
Explanation: Tip number 2 best answers this detail question. The tip recommends that
those who drink whole milk gradually switch to fat-free milk. Since the question asks about
ways to reduce saturated fat and calories, using skim milk in the place of water does not
address the issue being raised.

14. A
Explanation: The author uses headings to organize the passage. While the headings are
bold print, such font is not used to organize the passage (i.e. notify the reader of what
information is forthcoming), but rather to draw the reader's eyes to the headings.

15. C
Explanation: Tip number 2 bests answers this detail question. Reduced fat milk contains 2%
fat.

16. B
Explanation: Statement I and Statement II are both true statements about calcium rich
foods. Canned fish, including salmon with bones, is recommended as a calcium rich food.
Cheese is mentioned as a lactose-free alternative within the milk group. Statement III is
false. According to the passage, condensed cream soups should be made with milk, not
water.

17. D
Explanation: The best choice for this question is choice (D). The other options would clarify
information for minor details within the passage and would provide little new information
for the reader. However, food recommendations for those who do not consume milk
products are listed under a separate heading, and lactose intolerance is the only reason
listed. The reader can deduce that this is a main idea in the passage and the definition of
"lactose intolerance" would help explain this main idea to the reader.

18. B
Explanation: The word *exacerbate* means "aggravate." To *implicate* is "to demonstrate involvement or assign blame." To *decondition* is "to weaken or diminish the conditioned response to a certain stimulus."

19. D
Explanation: The word *repugnant* means "offensive, especially to the senses or the morals." The word *destructive* means "causing damage, injury, or loss." *Selective* means "choosy or capable of making a thoughtful choice." *Collective* means "combined or grouped together to form a whole."

20. A
Explanation: The word *compensatory* means "offsetting." *Defensive* means "protective" or "intending to repel an attack." *Untoward* means "unfavorable, improper, or unfortunate." *Confused* means "perplexed or bewildered."

21. B
Explanation: The best description for the word *flaccid* is "limp." The word *defended* means "driven danger away from." The word *slender* means "thin or skinny, but not to the extent of being unhealthy." The word *outdated* describes "something that has become irrelevant with age."

22. C
Explanation: The word *belligerent* means "pugnacious." *Pugnacious* means "ready to fight." The word *retired* means "withdrawn from business." The word *sardonic* means "mocking or sneering." The word *acclimated* means "used to or accustomed to."

23. A
Explanation: The best definition of the word *insidious* is "stealthy." The words *collapsed* and *new* have no innate relationship to the word *insidious*.

24. C
Explanation: The first paragraph states that the main purpose of DST it to make better use of daylight.

25. A
Explanation: Energy conservation is discussed as a possible benefit of DST, not a negative effect of it.

26. D
Explanation: The first paragraph states that DST involves setting clocks forward one hour in the spring and one hour backward in the fall.

27. D
Explanation: The sixth paragraph notes that DST is observed in only some regions of Brazil.

28. C
Explanation: If $30,000,000 is gained over 7 weeks, each week has a gain of 1/7 of that, or $4,200,000.

29. C

Explanation: Since both authors are explaining in the passages how the same story may come to be in different cultures, it is clear they both accept that there are often common elements in fairy tales from different cultures.

30. A

Explanation: The author of Passage 2 claims that the essence and nature of fairy tales is their representation of basic human experience. It is this assertion that leads the author to believe that the same story could develop independently in different places.

31. D

Explanation: The author does not mention the movement of food in the passage.

32. B

Explanation: The author never mentions witches in the passage.

33. A

Explanation: The passage suggests that spelunking is an outdoorsy, family adventure, then goes on to describe the adventure of going to a cave. If you do not already know that spelunking is another word for caving, you can infer this information based on reading the passage.

34. B

Explanation: The article's style is not technical or scientific in the least. It is a simple and lighthearted article about something a family could do together. It is adventurous, but *Adventures for Men* is not a good choice since the fun is for the whole family. *Mud Magazine* might have been the next best choice, but *Family Fun Days* is clearly better. Your job is to choose the best choice of the options given.

35. C

Explanation: Although it never specifically addresses the babysitter, the directions are clearly instructions for how to take care of a little girl. A mother or father would not need this information written down in such detail, but a babysitter might. You can infer the answer in this case.

36. D

Explanation: You cannot assume gender, and the note never indicates whether the writer is male or female. You can tell that the writer is the main caretaker of the child in question, so "parent" is the best choice in this case. A teacher or nurse might be able to write such a note, but parent is probably more likely, making it the best choice.

37. B

Explanation: The information in the passage lets you know that only the serving team can score. This rule is different in different leagues, so it is important to read the passage instead of going by what you know from your own life.

38. D
Explanation: Although any number of people could play in a volleyball game, the passage mentions that the entire class could participate in a game. Do all of them have to participate? No. But that wasn't the question.

39. A
Explanation: The referee might yell any number of things, but only "side out" is mentioned in the passage.

40. C
Explanation: In volleyball, all that is needed in terms of equipment is a ball and a net. Answer choice E, 15 points, is the number of points needed to win.

Mathematics Answer Explanations

1. B
Explanation: Multiply $120 by 24 months (a full two years) to get $2880. Add the thousand dollars for the down payment to get $3880. Find the difference between the entire amount all at once ($2600) and the amount pain in the plan ($3800). To find the difference, you subtract. The difference shows that $1280 more is paid with the installment plan.

2. C
Explanation: $29 + r = 420$
$29 + r - 29 = 420 - 29$
$r = 391$

3. C
Explanation: To solve, find the sum. $35\% + 4\% = 39\%$

4. C
Explanation: Electronics sales $= x$
$x = 35 + (-2) + (-1) + (+6) + (-1) + (+2)$
$x = (35 + 6 + 2) + (-2 + (-1) + (-1))$
$x = (43) + (-4)$
$x = 39$

5. B
Explanation: Add to solve. The height of the window from the floor is not needed in this equation. It is extra information. You only need to add the heights of the two bookcases. Change the fractions so that they have a common denominator. After you add, simply the fraction.
$14\frac{1}{2} + 8\frac{3}{4}$
$= 14\ 2/4 + 8\frac{3}{4}$
$= 22\ 5/4$
$= 23\frac{1}{4}$

6. B

Explanatioin: $y = x + 5$, and you were told that $x = -3$. Fill in the missing information for x, then solve.

$y = (-3) + 5$

$y = 2$

7. D

Explanation: Think of the numbers as they would be on a number line to place them in the correct order.

8. C

Explanation: In this problem, if you do not know how to solve, try filling in the answer choices to see which one checks out. Many math problems may be solved by a guess and check method when you have a selection of answer choices.

$27 - x = -5$

$x = 32$

9. A

Explanation: Add the numbers with x together, as follows: $5x + 4x = 9x$

Add the y numbers, as follows: $-2y + y = -y$

Put the x and y numbers back into the same equation: $9x - y$.

10. B

Explanation: To solve, line up the like terms, as follows:

$$
\begin{array}{r}
3x^2 + x + 3 \\
+ \quad 8x^2 + 5x + 16 \\
\hline
11x^2 + 6x + 19
\end{array}
$$

11. C

Explanation: To find perimeter, add the sides.

12. B

Explanation: 410 ml x 4 containers = 1640 ml

Change to liters: $1640 \div 1000 = 1.64$

Add the liter that was already in the pot: $1.64 + 1 = 2.64$ liters

13. D

Explanation: Snappy Twisters are the only ones that fall into the criteria listed in the question. The use of the words "no more than" is important to notice.

14. D

Explanation: Find the common denominator for the two fractions so that you can compare them. You can use the common denominator of 45, as follows:

$2/5 = 18/45$

$4/9 = 20/45$

Look at the numerators: 18 and 20. The number halfway between them is 19, so the answer is 19/45

15. A

Explanation: The fraction of ½ is the same as 50%. None of the other fractions are equal to that.

16. C

Explanation: $10\sqrt{6} \neq 6\sqrt{10}$.

$$36 = 6^2 \neq 6\sqrt{10}$$
$$\sqrt{600} = \sqrt{6 \cdot 100} = 10\sqrt{6} \neq 6\sqrt{10}$$
$$\sqrt{6} \neq 6\sqrt{10}$$
$$10\sqrt{6} \neq 6\sqrt{10}$$

17. C

Explanation: The expression 2^{-3} is equivalent to $\dfrac{1}{2^3}$, and since $2^3 = 8$, it is equivalent to

1/8.

a. $\dfrac{1}{4} = 2^{-2}$

b. $\dfrac{1}{12} \neq \dfrac{1}{8}$

d. $\dfrac{1}{16} = 2^{-4}$

18. B

Explanation: The value of the fraction $\dfrac{7}{5}$ can be evaluated by dividing 7 by 5, which yields

1.4. The average of 1.4 and 1.4 is $\dfrac{1.4 + 1.4}{2} = 1.4$.

19. D

Explanation: The product of x and $\dfrac{1}{x}$ is $\dfrac{1}{x} \times x = \dfrac{x}{x} = 1$. The expression x^{-1} is equivalent to

$\dfrac{1}{x}$. Thus, both B and C are correct.

A. $(x-1) \times x = x^2 - x \neq 1$

d. $x^2 \times x = x^3$, which is only equal to 1 if $x = 1$.

20. C

Explanation: The total distance traveled was 8 + 3.6 = 11.6 miles. The first 1/5th of a mile is charged at the higher rate. Since 1/5th = 0.2, the remainder of the trip is 11.4 miles. Thus the fare for the distance traveled is computed as $5.50 + 5 \times 11.4 \times \$1.50 = \$91$. To this the charge for waiting time must be added, which is simply 9 x 20¢ = 180¢ = $1.80. Finally, add the two charges, $91 + $1.80 = $92.80.

21. D

Explanation: Each term of each expression in parentheses must be multiplied by each term in the other. Thus for D, $(x+3)(3x-5) = 3x^2 + 9x - 5x - 15 = 3x^2 + 4x - 15$

a. $(x-3)(x+5) = x^2 - 3x + 5x - 15 = x^2 + 2x - 15 \neq 3x^2 + 4x - 15$

b. $(x+5)(3+x^2) = 3x + 15 + x^3 + 5x^2 \neq 3x^2 + 4x - 15$

c. $x(3x+4-15) = 3x^2 + 4x - 15x = 3x^2 - 11x \neq 3x^2 + 4x - 15$

22. B

Explanation: First determine the proportion of students in Grade 5. Since the total number of students is 180, this proportion is $\dfrac{36}{180} = 0.2$, or 20%. Then determine the same proportion of the total prizes, which is 20% of twenty, or $0.2 \times 20 = 4$.

a. $5 \neq 0.2 \times 20$

c. $7 \neq 0.2 \times 20$

d. $3 \neq 0.2 \times 20$

23. B

Explanation: A prime number is a natural, positive, non-zero number which can be factored only by itself and by 1. This is the case for 11.

a. 15 = 5 x 3, and thus is not a prime number.

c. 33 = 11 x 3, and thus is not a prime number.

d. 4 = 2 x 2, and thus is not a prime number.

24. A

Explanation: From the starting expression, compute:

$3(\dfrac{6x-3}{3}) - 3(9x+9) = 3(2x-1) - 27x - 27 = 6x - 3 - 27x - 27 = -21x - 30 = -3(7x+10)$

b. $-3x + 6 \neq 3(\dfrac{6x-3}{3}) - 3(9x+9)$

c. $(x+3)(x-3) = x^2 + 3x - 3x - 9 = x^2 - 9 \neq 3(\dfrac{6x-3}{3}) - 3(9x+9)$

d. $3x^2 - 9 \neq 3(\dfrac{6x-3}{3}) - 3(9x+9)$

25. B

Explanation: Compute as follows: $(3 - 2 \times 2)^2 = (3-4)^2 = (-1)^2 = 1$.

26. A

Explanation: Each glass of lemonade costs 10¢, or $0.10, so that g glasses will cost $g \times \$0.10$. To this, add Bob's fixed cost of $45, giving the expression in A.

27. c.
Explanation: Evaluate as follows:

$$(3x^{-2})^3 = 3^3 \times (x^{-2})^3 = 27 \times (\frac{1}{x^2})^3 = 27 \times \frac{1}{x^8} = 27x^{-8}$$

28. D
Explanation: Let P_A = the price of truck A and P_B that of truck b. Similarly let M_A and M_B represent the gas mileage obtained by each truck. The total cost of driving a truck n miles is

$$C = P + n \times \frac{\$4}{M}$$

To determine the break-even mileage, set the two cost equations equal to one another and solve for n:

$$P_A + n \times \frac{\$4}{M_A} = P_B + n \times \frac{\$4}{M_B}$$

$$n \times \left(\frac{\$4}{M_A} - \frac{\$4}{M_B} \right) = P_B - P_A$$

$$n = \frac{P_B - P_A}{\left(\frac{\$4}{M_A} - \frac{\$4}{M_B} \right)}$$

Plugging in the given values:

$$n = \frac{650 - 450}{\left(\frac{4}{25} - \frac{4}{35} \right)} = \frac{200}{\left(\frac{28}{175} - \frac{20}{175} \right)} = \frac{200}{\left(\frac{8}{175} \right)} = 4375 \text{ miles.}$$

29. C
Explanation: Rearranging the equation gives
$3(x+4) = 15(x-5)$, which is equivalent to
$15x - 3x = 12 + 75$, or
$12x = 87$, and solving for x,
$x = \frac{87}{12} = \frac{29}{4}.$

30. D
Explanation: The product *(a)(a)(a)(a)(a)* is defined as *a* to the fifth power.

31. D
Explanation: There are two ways to solve this problem: either convert meters to centimeters and then use the conversion factor in the table to convert centimeters to inches, or else use the table to convert meters to yards, and then convert to inches.

In the first instance, recall that there are 100 centimeters in a meter (*centi* means "hundredth"). Therefore $19m = 1900cm = (\frac{1900}{2.54}) = 748$ inches.

In the second instance, recall that there are 36 inches in a yard, therefore
$19m = 19 \times 1.094 = 20.786yd = 20.786 \times 36 = 748$ inches.

Proportions are commonly used for conversions. After converting meters to centimeters set up proportions to solve for an unknown variable, x.

$$\frac{1900 \text{ cm}}{x \text{ in.}} = \frac{2.54 \text{ cm}}{1 \text{ in}}$$ Cross multiply.

$1900 = 2.54x$ Divide each side by 2.54 to solve for x.

$x = 748$

32. A

Explanation: The mode is the number that appears most often in a set of data. If no item appears most often, then the data set has no mode. In this case, Kyle achieved one hit a total of three times, two hits twice, three hits once, and four hits once. One hit occurred the most times, therefore the mode of the data set is 1.

33. B

Explanation: The mean, or average, is the sum of the numbers in a data set divided by the total number of items. This data set contains seven items, one for each day of the week. The total number of hits that Kyle had during the week is the sum of the numbers in the right-hand column, or 14. This gives: $Mean = \dfrac{14}{7} = 2$.

34. D

Explanation: To multiply two binomials, use the FOIL method. FOIL stands for First, Outside, Inside, Last. When multiplying each pair of terms, remember to multiply the coefficients, then add the exponents of each separate variable. So the product of the First terms is $2a^2b \cdot 3a^3b = 6a^5b^2$. The product of the Outside terms is $2a^2b \cdot 4c = 8a^2bc$. The product of the Inside terms is $-3c^3 \cdot 3a^3b = -9a^3bc^3$. The product of the Last terms is $-3c^3 \cdot 4c = -12c^4$. The final answer is simply the sum of these four products.

35. D

Explanation: To find the percentage, divide the number of doctors in City X (74) by the total staff in City X (250), then multiply by 100. So we have $(74 \div 200) \times 100 = 29.8$ percent, which rounds up to 30.

36. A

Explanation: Because there is only one employee in City Y with more than 5 complaints, and we know that that employee is a speech pathologist, there can be no doctors with more than 5 complaints.

37. C

Explanation: To find each percentage, divide the first number by the second number, then multiply by 100. So the percentage in answer A is $(50 \div 250) \times 100 = 20$, the percentage in answer B is $(57 \div 250) \times 100 = 22.8$, the percentage in answer C is $[(74 + 55) \div 433] \times 100 = (129 \div 433) \times 100 = 29.8$, the percentage in answer D is $(21 \div 183) \times 100 = 11.5$, and the percentage in answer E is $(5 \div 183) \times 100 = 2.7$.

38. B
Explanation: There are 37 Caucasian staff members in City Y. If we subtract this from the number of employees with 5-10 years of service in City Y (41), we see that 4 of those staff members must be non-Caucasian.

39 B
Explanation: The percentage of female staff members in City Y is (90 ÷ 183) × 100 = 49.2. In City X, it is (97 ÷ 250) × 100 = 38.8. Subtracting, we see that the difference between these percentages is approximately 10.

40. B
Explanation: The percentage of staff members with zero complaints in City X is (202 ÷ 250) × 100 = 80.8. In City Y, the percentage is (161 ÷ 183) × 100 = 88.0.

41. D
Explanation: $-4x + 8 \geq 48$
To solve for x, first isolate the variable.
$-4x \geq 48 - 8$
$-4x \geq 40$
Then, divide both sides by -4 to solve for x.
When an inequality is divided by a negative number, the sign must change directions.
$-4x/-4 \geq 40/-4$
$x \leq -10$

42. D
Explanation: Integers include all positive and negative whole numbers and the number zero. The product of three integers must be an integer, so you can eliminate any answer choice that is not a whole number: choices (A) and (C). The product of two even integers is even. The product of even and odd integers is even. The only even choice is 24.

43. C
Explanation: Divide the mg the child should receive by the number of mg in 0.8 ml to determine how many 0.8 ml doses the child should receive: 240 ÷ 80 = 3. Multiply the number of doses by 0.8 to determine how many ml the child should receive: 3 X 0.8 = 2.4 ml

44. B
Explanation: The chart indicates that each x value must be tripled to equal the corresponding y value, so $y = 3x$. One way you can determine this is by plugging corresponding pairs of x and y into the answer choices.

45. D
Explanation: Use the following proportion: $\dfrac{1 \text{ in.}}{45 \text{ miles}} = \dfrac{3.2 \text{ inches}}{x \text{ miles}}$
Cross multiply: $x = (45)(3.2) = 144$

Science Answer Explanations

1. C
Explanation: A normal sperm must contain one of each of the human chromosome pairs. There are 23 chromosome pairs in all. Twenty-two of these are *autosomal* chromosomes, which do not play a role in determining gender. The remaining pair consists of either two X chromosomes in the case of a female, or of an X and a Y chromosome in the case of a male. Therefore, a normal sperm cell will contain 22 autosomal chromosomes and either an X or a Y chromosome, but not both.

2. B
Explanatioin: Oogenesis is the process that gives rise to the ovum, or egg, in mammals. The oocyte is the immature egg cell in the ovary. In humans, one oocyte matures during each menstrual cycle. It develops first into an intermediate form called the ootid, and eventually into an ovum. The prefix *oo-* is derived from Greek, and means "egg."

3. A
Explanation: In an oxidation reaction, an oxidizing agent gains electrons from a reducing agent. By contributing electrons, the reducing agent reduces (makes more negative) the charge on the oxidizer. In the car battery, reduction of the positively-charged anode provides electrons, which then flow to the cathode, where an oxidation takes place. In an oxidation, an oxidizing agent increases (makes more positive) the charge on a reducer. In this way, the extra electrons in the negatively charged cathode are neutralized by the surrounding oxidizing agent.

4. A
Explanation: The digestion of starch begins with its exposure to the enzyme amylase, which is present in the saliva. Amylase attacks the glycosidic bonds in starch, cleaving them to release sugars. This is the reason why some starchy foods may taste sweet if they are chewed extensively. Another form of amylase is produced by the pancreas, and continues the digestion of starches in the upper intestine. The di- and tri-saccharides, which are the initial products of this digestion, are eventually converted to glucose, a monosaccharide that is easily absorbed through the intestinal wall.

5. B
Explanation: The cell body, containing the nucleus, is the control center of the cell and the site of its metabolic activity. Dendrites, which extend from this cell body, receive signals from other cells in the form of neurotransmitters. This triggers an electrical impulse, which travels down the axon to the next cell on the route of the signal. At the end of the axon, neurotransmitters are again released, cross the synapse, and act upon the following cell.

6. C
Explanation: The pulmonary artery carries oxygen-depleted blood from the heart to the lungs, where CO_2 is released and the supply of oxygen is replenished. This blood then returns to the heart through the pulmonary artery, and is carried through the aorta and a series of branching arteries to the capillaries, where the bulk of gas exchange with the tissues occurs. Oxygen-depleted blood returns to the heart through branching veins (the femoral veins bring it from the legs) into the vena cava, which carries it again to the heart.

Since the pulmonary artery is the last step before replenishment of the blood's oxygen content, it contains the blood which is the most oxygen depleted.

7. D
Explanation: A tsunami, sometimes referred to as a tidal wave, is a large wave or series of waves caused by the displacement of a large volume of water. While the most common cause is an earthquake, large landslides (either falling into the sea or taking place under water) or explosive volcanic action may also result in a tsunami. Tsunamis take the appearance of very high, sustained tides, and may move water very far inland. Large storms, such as cyclones or hurricanes, may also displace great quantities of water, causing a high tide known as a storm surge that also resembles a tsunami.

8. D
Explanation: All living organisms on Earth utilize the same triplet genetic code, in which a three-nucleotide sequence called a codon provides information corresponding to a particular amino acid to be added to a protein. In contrast, many organisms, especially certain types of bacteria, do not use oxygen. These organisms live in oxygen-poor environments, and may produce energy through fermentation. Other organisms may live in dark environments, such as in caves or deep underground. Many organisms reproduce asexually by budding or self-fertilization, and only the most evolutionarily-advanced organisms make use of neurotransmitters in their nervous systems.

9. C
Explanation: Both cannonballs will be subject to a vertical acceleration due to the force of gravity. Although there is an additional horizontal component to the velocity of cannonball A, its vertical velocity will be the same. In each case, the height of the object at time t seconds will be $h = -\frac{1}{2}t^2 + 20$.

10. B
Explanation: It is impossible for an *AaBb* organism to have the *aa* combination in the gametes. It is impossible for each letter to be used more than one time, so it would be impossible for the lowercase *a* to appear twice in the gametes. It would be possible, however, for *Aa* to appear in the gametes, since there is one uppercase *A* and one lowercase *a*. Gametes are the cells involved in sexual reproduction. They are germ cells.

11. B
Explanation: Water stabilizes the temperature of living things. The ability of warm-blooded animals, including human beings, to maintain a constant internal temperature is known as *homeostasis*. Homeostasis depends on the presence of water in the body. Water tends to minimize changes in temperature because it takes a while to heat up or cool down. When the human body gets warm, the blood vessels dilate and blood moves away from the torso and toward the extremities. When the body gets cold, blood concentrates in the torso. This is the reason why hands and feet tend to get especially cold in cold weather. The exam will require you to understand the basic processes of the human body.

12. B
Explanation: Oxygen is not one of the products of the Krebs cycle. The *Krebs cycle* is the second stage of cellular respiration. In this stage, a sequence of reactions converts pyruvic

acid into carbon dioxide. This stage of cellular respiration produces the phosphate compounds that provide most of the energy for the cell. The Krebs cycle is also known as the citric acid cycle or the tricarboxylic acid cycle. The exam may require you to know all stages of cellular respiration: the process in which a plant cell converts carbon dioxide into oxygen.

13. C
Explanation: The sugar and phosphate in DNA are connected by covalent bonds. A *covalent bond* is formed when atoms share electrons. It is very common for atoms to share pairs of electrons. An *ionic bond* is created when one or more electrons are transferred between atoms. *Ionic bonds*, also known as *electrovalent bonds*, are formed between ions with opposite charges. There is no such thing as an *overt bond* in chemistry. The exam will require you to understand and have some examples of these different types of bonds.

14. A
Explanation: The second part of an organism's scientific name is its species. The system of naming species is called binomial nomenclature. The first name is the *genus*, and the second name is the *species*. In binomial nomenclature, species is the most specific designation. This system enables the same name to be used all around the world, so that scientists can communicate with one another. Genus and species are just two of the categories in biological classification, otherwise known as taxonomy. The levels of classification, from most general to most specific, are kingdom, phylum, class, order, family, genus, and species. As you can see, binomial nomenclature only includes the two most specific categories.

15. C
Explanation: Prokaryotic cells do not contain a nucleus. A *prokaryote* is simply a single-celled organism without a nucleus. It is difficult to identify the structures of a prokaryotic cell, even with a microscope. These cells are usually shaped like a rod, a sphere, or a spiral. A *eukaryote* is an organism containing cells with nuclei. Bacterial cells are prokaryotes, but since there are other kinds of prokaryotes, *bacteria* cannot be the correct answer to this question. *Cancer* cells are malignant, atypical cells that reproduce to the detriment of the organism in which they are located.

16. A
Explanation: Liquid is the densest form of water. Water can exist in three states, depending on temperature. Ranging from coldest to hottest, these states are solid, liquid, and gaseous—or ice, water, and steam. Water freezes at zero degrees Celsius. Although the solidity of ice might lead one to believe that it is the densest form of water, water actually expands about nine percent when it is frozen. This is the reason why ice will float in water. Steam is the least dense form of water.

17. B
Explanatioin: The oxidation number of the hydrogen in CaH_2 is –1. The oxidation number is the positive or negative charge of a monoatomic ion. In other words, the oxidation number is the numerical charge on an ion. An ion is a charged version of an element. Oxidation number is often referred to as oxidation state. Oxidation number is sometimes used to describe the number of electrons that must be added or removed from an atom in order to convert the atom to its elemental form.

18. C

Explanatioin: CH could be an empirical formula. An empirical formula is the smallest expression of a chemical formula. To be empirical, a formula must be incapable of being reduced. For this reason, answer choices A, B, and D are incorrect, as they could all be reduced to a simpler form. Note that empirical formulas are not the same as compounds, which do not have to be irreducible. Two compounds can have the same empirical formula but different molecular formulas. The molecular formula is the actual number of atoms in the molecule.

19. A

Explanation: A limiting reactant is entirely used up by the chemical reaction. Limiting reactants control the extent of the reaction and determine the quantity of the product. A reducing agent is a substance that reduces the amount of another substance by losing electrons. A reagent is any substance used in a chemical reaction. Some of the most common reagents in the laboratory are sodium hydroxide and hydrochloric acid. The behavior and properties of these substances are known, so they can be effectively used to produce predictable reactions in an experiment.

20. B

Explanation: The horizontal rows of the periodic table are called periods. The vertical columns of the periodic table are known as groups or families. All of the elements in a group have similar properties. The relationships between the elements in each period are similar as you move from left to right. The periodic table was developed by Dmitri Mendeleev to organize the known elements according to their similarities. New elements can be added to the periodic table without necessitating a redesign.

21. C

Explanation: The mass of 7.35 mol water is 132 grams. You should be able to find the mass of various chemical compounds when you are given the number of mols. The information required to perform this function is included on the periodic table. To solve this problem, find the molecular mass of water by finding the respective weights of hydrogen and oxygen. Remember that water contains two hydrogen molecules and one oxygen molecule. The molecular mass of hydrogen is roughly 1, and the molecular mass of oxygen is roughly 16. A molecule of water, then, has approximately 18 grams of mass. Multiply this by 7.35 mol, and you will obtain the answer 132.3, which is closest to answer choice c.

22. B

Explanation: 119°K is equivalent to –154 degrees Celsius. It is likely that you will have to perform at least one temperature conversion on the exam. To convert degrees Kelvin to degrees Celsius, simply subtract 273. To convert degrees Celsius to degrees Kelvin, simply add 273. To convert degrees Kelvin into degrees Fahrenheit, multiply by 9/5 and subtract 460. To convert degrees Fahrenheit to degrees Kelvin, add 460 and then multiply by 5/9. To convert degrees Celsius to degrees Fahrenheit, multiply by 9/5 and then add 32. To convert degrees Fahrenheit to degrees Celsius, subtract 32 and then multiply by 5/9.

23. A

Explanation: There are four different types of tissue in the human body: epithelial, connective, muscle, and nerve. *Epithelial* tissue lines the internal and external surfaces of the body. It is like a sheet, consisting of squamous, cuboidal, and columnar cells. They can expand and contract, like on the inner lining of the bladder. *Connective* tissue provides the

- 113 -

structure of the body, as well as the links between various body parts. Tendons, ligaments, cartilage, and bone are all examples of connective tissue. *Muscle* tissue is composed of tiny fibers, which contract to move the skeleton. There are three types of muscle tissue: smooth, cardiac, and skeletal. *Nerve* tissue makes up the nervous system; it is composed of nerve cells, nerve fibers, neuroglia, and dendrites.

24. B
Explanation: The epidermis is the outermost layer of skin. The thickness of this layer of skin varies over different parts of the body. For instance, the epidermis on the eyelids is very thin, while the epidermis over the soles of the feet is much thicker. The dermis lies directly beneath the epidermis. It is composed of collagen, elastic tissue, and reticular fibers. Beneath the dermis lies the subcutaneous tissue, which consists of fat, blood vessels, and nerves. The subcutaneous tissue contributes to the regulation of body temperature. The hypodermis is the layer of cells underneath the dermis; it is generally considered to be a part of the subcutaneous tissue.

25. D
Explanation: Of the given structures, veins have the lowest blood pressure. *Veins* carry oxygen-poor blood from the outlying parts of the body to the heart. An *artery* carries oxygen-rich blood from the heart to the peripheral parts of the body. An *arteriole* extends from an artery to a capillary. A *venule* is a tiny vein that extends from a capillary to a larger vein.

26. C
Explanataion: Of the four heart chambers, the left ventricle is the most muscular. When it contracts, it pushes blood out to the organs and extremities of the body. The right ventricle pushes blood into the lungs. The atria, on the other hand, receive blood from the outlying parts of the body and transport it into the ventricles. The basic process works as follows: Oxygen-poor blood fills the right atrium and is pumped into the right ventricle, from which it is pumped into the pulmonary artery and on to the lungs. In the lungs, this blood is oxygenated. The blood then reenters the heart at the left atrium, which when full pumps into the left ventricle. When the left ventricle is full, blood is pushed into the aorta and on to the organs and extremities of the body.

27. A
Explanation: The *cerebrum* is the part of the brain that interprets sensory information. It is the largest part of the brain. The cerebrum is divided into two hemispheres, connected by a thin band of tissue called the corpus callosum. The *cerebellum* is positioned at the back of the head, between the brain stem and the cerebrum. It controls both voluntary and involuntary movements. The *medulla oblongata* forms the base of the brain. This part of the brain is responsible for blood flow and breathing, among other things.

28. C
Explanation: *Collagen* is the protein produced by cartilage. Bone, tendon, and cartilage are all mainly composed of collagen. *Actin* and *myosin* are the proteins responsible for muscle contractions. Actin makes up the thinner fibers in muscle tissue, while myosin makes up the thicker fibers. Myosin is the most numerous cell protein in human muscle. *Estrogen* is one of the steroid hormones produced mainly by the ovaries. Estrogen motivates the menstrual cycle and the development of female sex characteristics.

29. C

Explanation: The parasympathetic nervous system is responsible for lowering the heart rate. It slows down the heart rate, dilates the blood vessels, and increases the secretions of the digestive system. The central nervous system is composed of the brain and the spinal cord. The sympathetic nervous system is a part of the autonomic nervous system; its role is to oppose the actions taken by the parasympathetic nervous system. So, the sympathetic nervous system accelerates the heart, contracts the blood vessels, and decreases the secretions of the digestive system.

30. A

Explanation: An adult inhales 500 mL of air in an average breath. Interestingly, humans can inhale about eight times as much air in a single breath as they do in an average breath. People tend to take a larger breath after making a larger inhalation. This is one reason that many breathing therapies, for instance those incorporated into yoga practice, focus on making a complete exhalation. The process of respiration is managed by the autonomic nervous system. The body requires a constant replenishing of oxygen, so even brief interruptions in respiration can be damaging or fatal.

English and Language Usage Answer Explanations

1. C

Explanation: In the original text, the word "would" is slang and adds nothing to the sentence. Answers B and D differ in meaning from the original.

2. D

Explanation: The hyphens clarify the meaning by showing that the entire three-word clause modifies the expression "food supply."

3. B

Explanation: By separating the modifying clause "in recent years," it clarifies the meaning of the sentence.

4. B

Explanation: The original does not specify who is referred to by the word "their," which is unnecessary. Answer D is is incorrect usage.

5. B

Explanation: The word "that" has already appeared ("you would think that...") and is redundant if used again here.

6. A

Explanation: None of the other spellings make sense in this usage.

7. A

Explanation: The percentage plainly refers to the population mentioned earlier in the sentence. All the other answers are redundant.

8. B

Explanation: Answer B which is the possessive of a plural noun. The original text offers the possessive of a singular noun, which is incorrect. The other answers are not possessives.

9. B
Explanation: Answer B is also the simplest. The word "still" in the original suggests that people will not buy expensive foods even if some other condition is met, but no such condition is specified. Therefore, the word is unnecessary and confusing.

10. B
Explanation: The word "your" in the original is slang usage. Answer C is incorrect because it is a plural, not a possessive.

11. D
Explanation: In this case, "too" means "also."

12. B
Explanation: The phrase is redundant since the word "theory" is included in the name "the paycheck cycle theory" which follows immediately afterwards in the sentence.

13. C
Explanation: The word "family" is used redundantly in the original sentence, and is easily replaced by a pronoun in this case.

14. C
Explanation: The hypothesis suggests the *existence* of a cycle that promotes weight gain. In the original, the word "that" makes the sentence nonsensical.

15. C
Explanation: The use of "would" in the original is slang. The author is saying that, if the paycheck cycle hypothesis is correct, the two causes of overweight are periodic food restriction and poor diet. Since there is some uncertainty here, C is a better choice than b.
16. C
Explanation: Answer C is the possessive of the plural noun "women."

17. C
Explanation: Answer C is a possessive. Answer D is technically correct, but it is common usage to use this expression as a collective noun, so that "porter's lodge" can describe a lodge for more than one porter.

18. C
Explanation: The other answers do not make sense.

19. D
Explanation: The original text's "accesses" requires a singular subject.

20. B
Explanation: Answer C changes the meaning, suggesting that the action is not performed every day, whereas the original text indicates that it occurs daily but that the time is indefinite.

21. A

Explanation: "Entryway" is the correct spelling.

22. B

Explanation: The phrase in the original is unnecessary, and is redundant as it repeats "only." The other answers are unnecessarily wordy.

23. C

Explanation: The original text splits the infinitive "to receive." Answers B and D imply that this happens all the time, whereas the text implies that it is an exceptional occurrence.

24. D

Explanation: Answer C repeats the word "even" and is redundant.

25. B

Explanation: The original text is phrased awkwardly, and answers C and D change the meaning.

26. B

Explanation: This provides a parallel construction between "morning" and "evening."

27. C

Explanation: The original seeks to imply that the guards are not effectively on watch, but the phrasing is awkward and makes no sense. Answer B is correctly spelled, but retains the awkward phrasing of the original.

28. D

Explanation: Since all the elements of the list contain verbs, this choice provides for parallel construction by also including the verb. Answer C is less desirable since the phrase "physically out of shape" is redundant.

29. B

Explanation: The other choices are unnecessarily wordy.

30. D

Explanation: Answer D most specifically explains what has been ineffective about the tactics of the guards. Answer C is vague.

31. D

Explanation: The word *our* makes the sentence grammatically correct. *Our* is the possessive case of *we*, In this case, our is being used as an attributive adjective. An adjective is a word that modifies (or describes) a noun. *Our* is called an attributive adjective because it is attributing (assigning) ownership of the screaming to a particular party, *us*. Answer choices A and D are in the first-person plural; answer choices B and C are in the third-person plural. Neither B nor C, however, is in the possessive case. The sentence could be effectively completed with *their*, but this choice is not available.

32. A

Explanation: The phrase *dog, who had* makes the sentence grammatically correct. To begin with, it is necessary for there to be a comma separating these two clauses, because the

- *117* -

second clause is nonrestrictive. A clause is considered nonrestrictive if it could not stand by itself and if the rest of the sentence would still make sense were it removed. If the portion of this sentence after the comma were removed, the sentence would be *Janet called her dog*. Obviously, this is still a coherent sentence. Also, *who* is used here instead of *which* because the antecedent, *dog*, has an identity and personality.

33. D
Explanation: The word *one* is used incorrectly in this sentence. Here, *one* is being used as a pronoun: a stand-in for some other noun. The problem is that it is unclear to what it is referring. The only possible reference for *one* is video store, and it does not make sense to say that "we should rent a video store." Most of the time, we would read this sentence and just assume that the author meant that we should rent a video. However, on the exam, you must be alert for unclear wording.

34. B
Explanation: The preposition *among* is not used correctly in the context of the sentence. In this case, the word *between* would be more appropriate. *Among* and *between* both mean "in the midst of some other things." However, *between* is used when there are only two other things, and *among* is used when there are more than two. For example, it would be correct to say "between first and second base" or "among several friends." In this sentence, the preposition *among* is inappropriate for describing placement amid "two treatment protocols."

35. B
Explanation: The part of the sentence "who says that…" is a parenthetical phrase about Richard Louv, not about the subject of the sentence. The "and who" is therefore incorrect, and the phrase needs to be set off from the sentence by a comma.

36. C
Explanation: The best answer is (C) because it best captures the logical connection of the sentences: the fear of abduction is the *reason* parents are afraid to let kids play in the woods.
37. D
Explanation: The sentence needs a subject. Answer (D) is the one that most clearly identifies a subject.

38. D
Explanation: The "this" logically must refer to child abduction. Although not stated explicitly, it is the only choice that could logically be described as "a terrible thing" and "very rare."

39. B
Explanation: Although the paragraph does not make its point explicitly, it clearly states that kids are spending too much time with video games and TV (being entertained by technology) and would be helped by more time getting their feet and hands dirty and touching things rather than just reading about them (having a +sensory experience of nature).

40. B

Explanation: You may already know that a conifer is a type of tree. If you do not know this, you can deduce the information based on the fact that the word is used in the description of the Giant Sequoia tree.

41. D

Explanation: In the first sentence, the passage states that *most* people think the Giant Sequoia is the largest organism. It goes on to explain that there are some people who do not agree.

42. C

Explanation: Look at lines 10 and 11 to find the answer. The passage explains that goldenrod flowers and aspen groves are connected with underground root systems, leading some people to believe that these organisms are bigger than Giant Sequoia trees.

43. D

Explanation: The passage gives the diameter of the tree at the bottom, but the diameter at the top is not given. You cannot assume the answer, so there is no way to know what the diameter is given the data in the passage.

44. C

Explanation: The word *closely* makes the sentence grammatically correct. Remember that an adjective is a word that describes a noun, while an adverb describes an adjective, a verb, or another adverb. In this sentence, you are looking for the right word to describe how the attendant *looked*. This means that you are looking for an adverb. Most of the time, adverbs end in *-ly*. On question 20, answer choices C and D both have this ending. Answer choice D, however, does not really make sense when substituted into the sentence.

45. A

Explanation: The phrase *more efficient* makes the sentence grammatically correct. Here, the author is attempting to describe a comparison between two things: the coal furnace and the woodstove. The comparative form of an adjective usually ends with *-er*: *taller, wiser, cleaner*, for example. In some cases, however, the word *more* is placed in front of the unchanged adjective. As a general rule, multisyllabic words are more likely to use the *more* construction than the *-er* construction. That is the case with *efficient*. Unfortunately, there is no easy rule for memorizing the comparative forms of common English adjectives. Reading is one way to develop a good eye for proper usage.

46. C

Explanation: The word *hungrily* makes the sentence grammatically correct. In order to answer this question, you must know the difference between an adjective and an adverb. An adjective modifies a noun. For instance, in the phrase *the delicious meatball, delicious* is an adjective. An adverb, on the other hand, modifies an adjective, a verb, or another adverb. In the phrase *walking quickly away, quickly* is an adverb. In the sentence for this question, it seems clear that the answer must modify the verb *eyed*. After all, it would not make much sense for the cheesecake to be hungry. This means that an adverb is required. The adverbial form of *hungry* is *hungrily*.

47. A

Explanation: The phrase *him or her* makes the sentence grammatically correct. In this case, we are looking for a word or words that can serve as the object of the preposition *for*. *She* and *he* are nominative forms, meaning that they can only be used as the subject of a sentence or a clause. *Them* can be the object of a preposition, but it is plural and, therefore, cannot correctly refer to the singular subject *a child*. (Incidentally, the use of *they* and *them* to refer to a singular subject is one of the most common grammatical errors, and will almost certainly appear in one or more questions on the exam.) For a similar reason, you cannot use *it* to refer to *a child*. The correct answer, then, is *him or her*.

48. C

Explanation: The phrase *she and I* makes the sentence grammatically correct. The blank needs to be filled by the subject of the sentence. The subject of a sentence or clause is the person, place, or thing that performs the verb. There are a couple of ways to determine that this sentence needs a subject. To begin with, the blank is at the beginning of the sentence, where the subject most often is found. Also, when you read the sentence, you will notice that it is unclear who went to the movies. Because you are looking for the subject, you need the nominative pronouns *she and I*.

49. C

Explanation: The word *effected* is not spelled correctly in the context of this sentence. In order to answer this question, you need to know the difference between *affect* and *effect*. The former is a verb and the latter is a noun. In other words, *affect* is something that you do and *effect* is something that is. In this sentence, the speaker is describing something that the prescription medication *did*. Therefore, the appropriate word is a verb. *Effect*, however, is a noun. For this reason, instead of *effected* the author should have used the word *affected*.

50. B

Explanation: The word *hear* is not spelled correctly in the context of this sentence. The speaker has mixed up the homophones *hear* and *here*. *Homophones* are words that sound the same but are spelled differently and have a different meaning. Homophones are not to be confused with *homonyms*, which are spelled the same but have a different meaning. In question 5, the author is trying to describe the place where the climate is; that is, he or she is describing the climate *here*. Unfortunately, the author uses the word *hear*, which is a verb meaning "to listen."

51. B

Explanation: The word *further* is not used correctly in the context of this sentence. Here, the word *farther* would be more appropriate. The distinction between *further* and *farther* is likely to appear in at least one question on the exam. For the purposes of the examination, you just need to know that *farther* can be used to describe physical distance, while *further* cannot. In this sentence, the speaker is describing a distance to be walked, which is a physical distance. For this reason, the word *further* is incorrect.

52. B

Explanation: The preposition *among* is not used correctly in the context of the sentence. In this case, the word *between* would be more appropriate. *Among* and *between* both mean "in the midst of some other things." However, *between* is used when there are only two other things, and *among* is used when there are more than two. For example, it would be correct to say "between first and second base" or "among several friends." In this sentence, the

- 120 -

preposition *among* is inappropriate for describing placement amid "two treatment protocols."

53. B
Explanation: To say something is sincere means that it is genuine or real. For example, saying someone showed sincere concern means that their concern was genuine, and not fake.

54. B
Explanation: Describing somebody as courteous implies that they are polite and well-mannered. Polite and courteous both convey the same meaning.

55. C
Explanation: If you say that you comprehend something, it is the same as saying you understand it. For example, saying you comprehend what another person is saying is the same as saying you understand them.